"Nurses' Voices

From the Northern Ireland Troubles

"Nurses' Voices

From the Northern Ireland Troubles

Personal accounts from the front line
edited by **Margaret Graham and Professor Jean Orr**

This book is dedicated to all nurses, midwives and health visitors who worked through the Northern Ireland Troubles and to those for whom they cared.

The History of Nursing Network, RCN Northern Ireland in association with RCN Publishing Company Limited

RCN Publishing Company Limited,
The Heights, 59–65 Lowlands Road,
Harrow-on-the-Hill,
Middlesex HA1 3AW

First published 2013
Second edition 2013
Published in paperback 2014

British Library Cataloguing in Publication Data. A catalogue record for this book is
available from the British Library.

Disclaimer

ISBN: 978 0 9574308 7 7 (hbk)
ISBN: 978 0 9574308 3 9 (pbk)
ISBN: 978 0 9574308 1 5 (ebk)

Cover background image: Shankill bomb, ©Press Association
Cover design by Wendy Dunbar, Dunbar Design
Designed by Angie Moyes and Ken McLoone
Typeset by Aptara, Inc.
Printed by Cambrian Printers

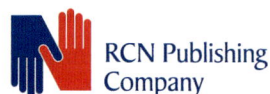

RCN Publishing
Company

The History of Nursing Network in Northern Ireland has gathered stories from nurses, midwives and health visitors who worked during the period of civil unrest in Northern Ireland from 1969 to the Belfast Agreement (1998).

These stories add to the untold stories of a community under strife and demonstrate the impact civil unrest had on nurses who were also part of the community they served.

This publication, made possible by a generous bequest from Dr Mona Grey, will ensure that the single prevailing message of all participants to "gather our stories before they are lost" will be a lasting testimony to them and all nurses who met challenges not seen outside of a war zone with such high standards of professionalism and humanity.

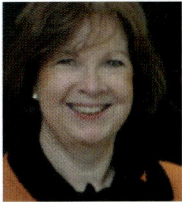

Margaret Graham

History of Nursing Network
RCN Northern Ireland
Book Project Leader

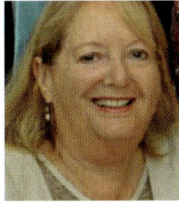

Professor Jean Orr

Queen's University Belfast
Story Editor

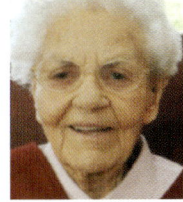

Dr Mona Grey

Fellow of the
Royal College of Nursing

"This brilliant book reflects on a time of dreadful loss and tragedy... today's nurses should read these first-hand accounts of what true care and compassion are really all about."

Mary Spinks, former Director of the Florence Nightingale Foundation

"These raw accounts of nursing, in situations that most of us will hopefully never face, make compelling reading. A gripping and brutally honest tapestry of dark days of conflict, yet enlivened by many flashes of humour."

John Adams, Senior Lecturer, Anglia University

"A fascinating window onto the Troubles and an important contribution to the social history of nursing."

Dr Marc Cornock, Lecturer in Law, The Open University

Contents

Dr Mona Grey MBE OBE FRCN

Nurses who tell their stories

Foreword

About the Northern Ireland conflict

'Blood on my Apron'

With grateful thanks to the late

Dr Mona Grey MBE OBE FRCN

The publication of this book has been made possible by a generous bequest made by Dr Mona Grey to the Royal College of Nursing (RCN).

Mona Grey was born in Rawalpindi, India in 1910, the year that Florence Nightingale died. She initially trained as a teacher in India, before returning to England where she was accepted for nurse training at the London Hospital. She excelled during her training and held posts as a Staff Nurse and a Ward Sister before being appointed Night Superintendent during the Second World War.

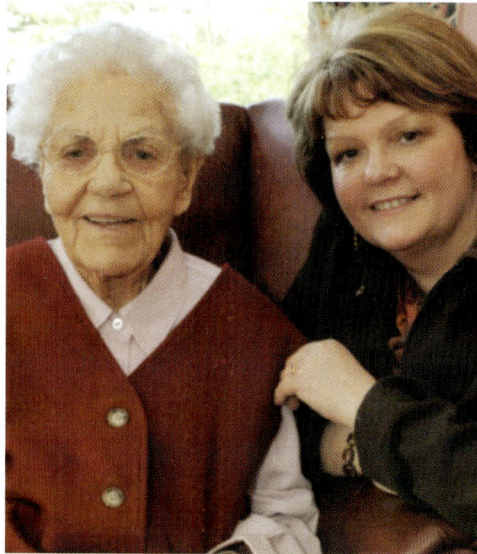

Above: Dr Mona Grey with Janice Smyth, Director, RCN Northern Ireland. Right: Dr Grey in the 1950s

The RCN established a branch in Belfast in 1925 with funding initially provided by the Nuffield Foundation. In 1946 Mona was appointed as the first salaried Secretary. Her primary task was to secure the financial future of the RCN in Northern Ireland, so she set up an Appeals Committee. Various social activities were organised and the target of £50,000 was well exceeded. The biggest fundraising events came from another passion of Mona's — a love of the performing arts.

In 1951, at the request of the Belfast Committee of the Festival of Britain, she wrote and produced a pageant —

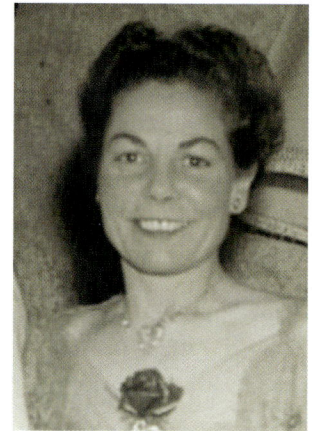

'A Cavalcade of Nursing'. As the opening event for the festival in Northern Ireland, this was very successful. Other plays and events followed, equally dramatic and financially beneficial.

Her appointment in 1960 as the first Chief Nursing Officer in the Department of Health and Social Services of Northern Ireland was further evidence of her commitment and nursing leadership. During this time she played a central role in restructuring the health service in Northern Ireland. Mona was awarded an MBE in 1952 for her services to nursing; an OBE in 1974 and an Honorary Degree from the University of Ulster in 1999. She was made a Fellow of the RCN in 2004.

Mona was a teacher, a nurse, a trade union leader, a civil servant and, in later years, a champion of the elderly. She died peacefully in 2009 at the age of 98, having led a full and productive life.

Nurses who tell their stories

Attracta Bradley
Ann Brown
Irene Brush
Geraldine Byers
Anne Patterson Campbell
Kathleen Canney
Kate Catney
Ursula Clifford
Sean Collins
Annie Courtney
Carolyn Crouchman
Maurice Devine
Ethel Dundas
Helen Dunwoody
Lorna Finlay
Catherine Gallagher
Jean Garland
Noelle Gormley
Deborah Graffin
Margaret Graham
Anne Grant
Edna Grant
Norma Grindle
John Hall
Eleanor Hayes
Reba Jackson
Laurie Jones
Margaret Kelly
Margaret Kerr
Lorna Liggett
Ann Little
Iris Loney
Garrett Martin

Marianne Moutray
Anne Murdock
Ann Murray
Orla McAlinden
Elizabeth McAlister
Margaret McCambridge
Margaret McCann
Mary McCullagh
Martha McEvoy
Isabelle McFarlane
Frances McMillan
Pamela McMillen
Sally McMulkin
Martelle McPartland
Miriam McReynolds
Jean Orr
Jane Packham
Sandra Peake
Vera Poots
Amy Pullman
Horace Reid
Maureen Reid
Kathleen Robb
Kathy Rowe
Tom Rush
Kathleen Slevin
Ruth Smith
Clare Smyth
Jenny Stevenson
Irene Symington
Joy Wallace
Eric Wilkinson
John Williams

The Royal College of Nursing congratulates the History of Nursing Network in Northern Ireland for gathering these stories from nurses across the province to create this book.
The accounts cover three decades of violence and are an important addition, not only to our local nursing history but to the wider national nursing history.
In particular the RCN thanks all participants who have so willingly contributed to this project.

Foreword

Some years ago the History of Nursing Network, RCN Northern Ireland was asked to consider gathering stories from nurses who had worked through the extended period of civil unrest commonly referred to as "the Troubles". This book is the result of that request and is a collection of previously untold stories from nurses directly involved in nursing, midwifery and health visiting during the period of conflict in Northern Ireland between August 1969 and the Belfast Agreement in 1998 and beyond. This was a time of almost unbroken civil unrest resulting in injuries from bombs and bullets not normally seen outside a war zone.

The History of Nursing Network, or what is popularly known as the 'History Group', has been active for many years. Composed mostly of retired nurses, an important aspect of its activities has been to ensure that local nursing history has its place within the national context. Thus for a number of years oral histories from retired nurses from across the province have been recorded. These taped records form part of the National RCN Archive in London.

When the History Group was asked to consider gathering stories for publication from nurses who had worked through the 30-odd years of the Troubles, it seemed a natural extension of its activities. As members reflected on their respective nursing careers during this period, it became obvious how events dominated the working and personal lives of nurses in all disciplines across Northern Ireland. The group realised that "the job had to be done". These stories had to be recorded properly and told before they were lost.

But where and how to start?
Much has already been written about the Troubles and their economic, political and

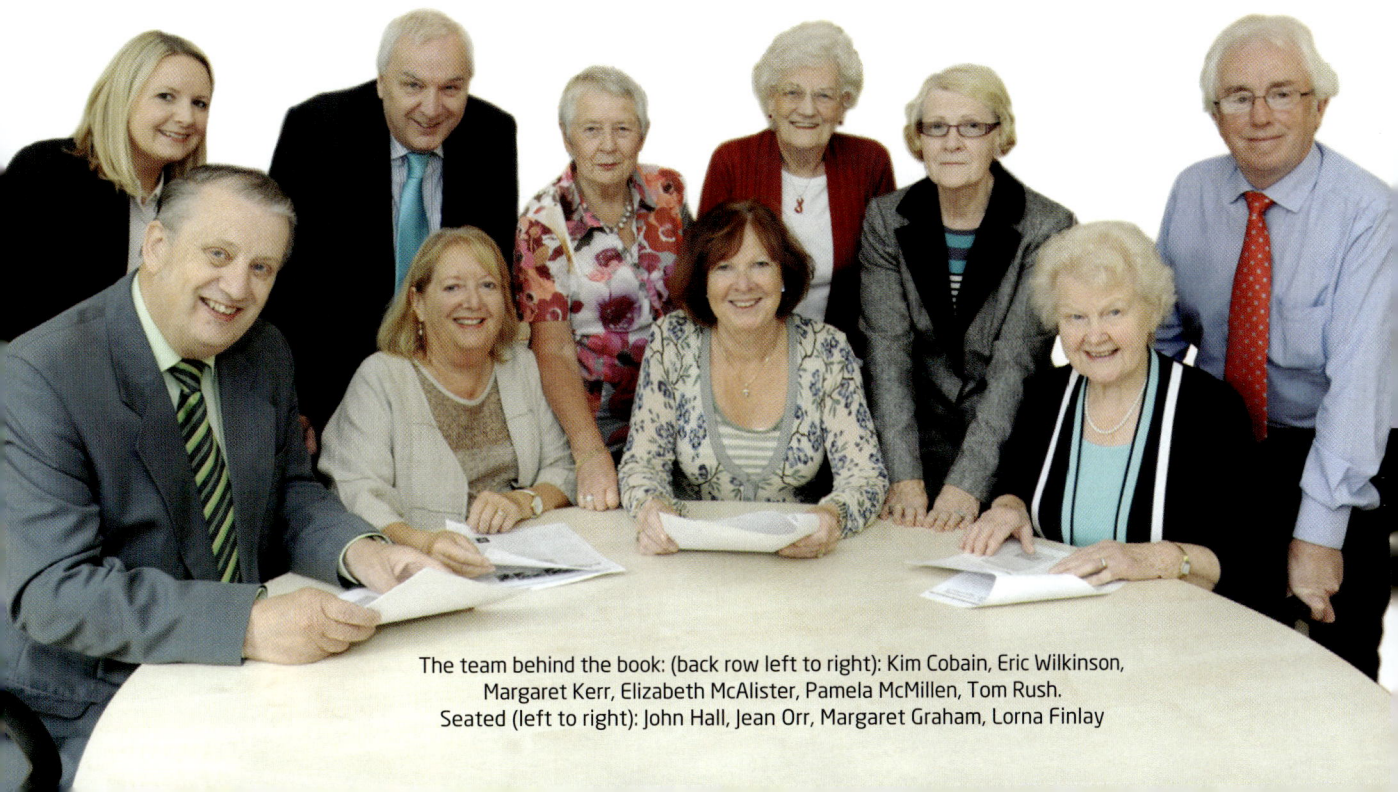

The team behind the book: (back row left to right): Kim Cobain, Eric Wilkinson, Margaret Kerr, Elizabeth McAlister, Pamela McMillen, Tom Rush. Seated (left to right): John Hall, Jean Orr, Margaret Graham, Lorna Finlay

social outcomes. Despite this wealth of coverage there has, to date, been no comprehensive account of nursing through this period.

In reality the Troubles did not start or finish on a particular date but there was an upsurge of violence in the year 1969 and this continued up to the Good Friday or Belfast Agreement in April 1998. Within the History Group there was a strong consensus to include some stories related to major events that happened after this period, such as the Omagh Bomb (August 1998) and disturbances at the annual Orange Order July marches at Drumcree Church, Portadown (1995-1998). By their scale and nature they fitted the tenor of the book.

The extraordinary very quickly became the ordinary. It became ordinary to deal with amputations, major burns and blast damage and many types of complex injuries to head, body and mind. Nurses working in the community often found themselves caught in crossfire or having to negotiate their way through barricades to visit families, give insulin or change a dressing. Those travelling in or out of work to hospitals and clinics had similar experiences. Some describe dark streets because all lights had been deliberately smashed. Others had to negotiate with paramilitaries to be allowed through barricades. Many walked along streets of rubble because there was no public

transport and often taxi drivers were hesitant to operate in troubled areas.

Given the historical background to the Northern Ireland conflict, nurses, as part of the community, could hold different loyalties and political aspirations. Sometimes in particularly stressful situations this caused tensions. However, as the Troubles continued, strongly held personal convictions became subservient to the needs of the patient whatever their background or circumstance.

From the outset, the aim of the History Group was to give some insight into nursing at all levels, all disciplines, in hospitals and in communities. In common with other health professionals, nurses were often in the front line, caring for their patients.

All the stories have been written by the individuals involved. Some have sent us their previously published stories. Many have admitted that the process was difficult but cathartic; bringing back painful memories of past events. We hope that this book will ensure that the single prevailing message of all participants – "to gather stories before they are lost" – will be a lasting testimony to all nurses who, being part of the community, met this challenge with professionalism and humanity.

The History of Nursing Network,
RCN Northern Ireland

About the Northern Ireland conflict

- Every day of the year marks the anniversary of someone's death as a result of conflict in and about Northern Ireland.[1]

- In 1971 the population of Northern Ireland was 1,536,065; in 1981 it was 1,488,077.[2]

- Between 1968 and 1998 some 3,725 people were killed as a result of the conflict.[3]

- Approximately 47,541 people were injured.[4]

- There were 36,923 shootings.[5]

- 16,209 bombings took place.[5]

- A total of 1,533 of the deaths as a result of the conflict were among people under the age of 25, and 257 of those killed were under the age of 18.[6]

- The largest age group among the dead were young people between 18 and 23 years, amounting to one quarter of those killed (898 people).[6]

- As of 1998, the largest group of victims of the conflict (54%) were civilians.[6]

- As of 1998, the largest group of those injured (68%) were civilians.[6]

References on page 189

Blood on my Apron

Blood, spreading out, ever-widening,
Like ripples caused by a stone thrown into a pond.
Rich, vibrant, ruby-red,
Staining the white cotton crispness
Of my starched apron.

Blood speaks of life,
But this blood spells death.

I have blood on my apron,
But you have blood on your hands.

Are there no other ways of settling disputes,
Except by bloodshed?

Will all this carnage never end?
Will we ever have peace?
Or will there always be blood on my apron?

Vera E Poots (née Hunniford)

A personal journey through the Troubles

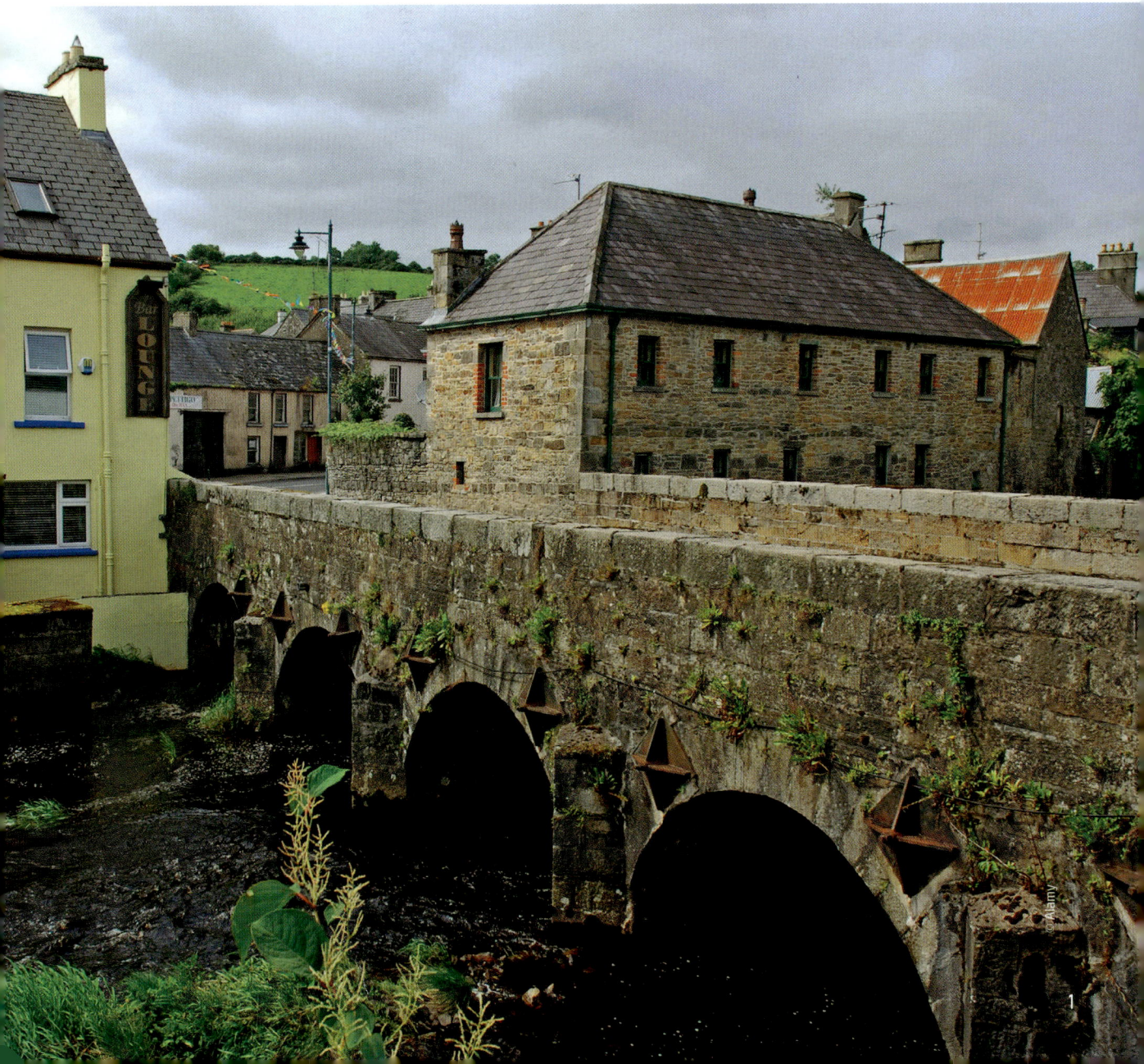

When the Troubles erupted in full force in 1969, any students or staff nurses just beginning their careers could not have foreseen that most of their working life would be dominated by the impact of prolonged civil unrest and violence.

Nurses who trained and worked in hospitals sited close to areas of intense conflict were the most likely to see casualties of punishment beatings, bombs and bullets. For those nurses who came from quiet communities untouched by the unrest, exposure to civil disturbances and casualties was a traumatic initiation.

The following story from a retired male staff nurse shows how an entire nursing career could span the duration of the Troubles…

In the course of a lifetime

❝I was born and reared on the Border's edge near a village called Pettigo. It nestles between the hills of South Donegal and North Fermanagh and sits astride the gently flowing River Termon which, in that part of the country, is effectively a national boundary.

The village only seemed to come alive in the summer months – at least for a few hours each day – when thousands of pilgrims made their way from all over Ireland via the village's equally sleepy railway station en route to St Patrick's Purgatory, an island on nearby Lough Derg. In the austere post-World War Two years of my childhood, television, and mains electricity, were not available. 'Céilidh' – visiting neighbours houses – was still very much part of the local culture.

It was on such visits to neighbours with my father that I first became aware of earlier conflicts. I would listen to old men recounting experiences of the 'War of Pettigo' in the summer of 1922 between the Crown Forces and the IRA. Sadly lives were lost on both sides. When I was about nine years of age, however, I had my first personal exposure to the unrest which was to become an enduring reality for all the people of Northern Ireland, but particularly those of us living near the Border.

The IRA's 1956-1962 campaign saw the stepping up of security. Fortification of police stations, sealing of cross-border roads, mobilisation of the Ulster Special Constabulary to guard strategic areas and deployment of armoured transport, mostly ex-army World War Two vehicles, brought a change to this normally quiet rural backwater. It was not apparent then, but on reflection it is amazing how the unfolding events did not deflect from the solidarity and friendliness of this predominantly farming community regardless of religion, political persuasion or on which side of the river the people resided. I recall no terrorist incidents in North West Fermanagh during that campaign.

Nurse training
In 1965 I moved to Omagh and started psychiatric nurse training. After obtaining my Registered Mental Nurse qualification and a period of 'staffing' in Tyrone &

Fermanagh Hospital, I was accepted for general training at the Royal Victoria Hospital (RVH) on 2 January 1970. New Troubles had started but few could have envisaged how these would affect the lives of every individual in the province, regardless of where they lived, or the effect it would have on casualty and healthcare provision.

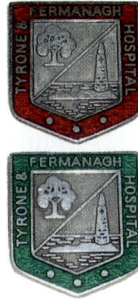

Initially my student placements brought me into direct contact with only a few victims of the Troubles. After a placement in orthopaedics and other areas I was moved to theatres. On my first night duty an army foot patrol of some seven or eight members was ambushed not far from the hospital. Several were brought to theatre where we removed low-velocity bullets and other shrapnel. Fortunately all the patrol survived, with the worst injury necessitating the amputation of a finger.

Less fortunate was another elderly male civilian who was shot in the forehead the same night. I recall a consultant neurosurgeon and team of theatre nurses working most of the night in an unsuccessful attempt to save his life. In all probability this team would become part of the innovative work in head injuries for which the RVH gained worldwide renown.

On another occasion as I was preparing to leave the hospital grounds I heard a burst of gunfire followed by shouting nearby. As soon as I considered it safe I went over in that direction and found a soldier badly wounded in the abdomen. With the assistance of a porter we were able to get

him to accident and emergency (A&E) on a trolley within minutes but, regrettably, I heard on the news later in the day that he had died from his wounds.

The other Troubles-related event in which I was involved was the aftermath of the explosion at McGurk's Bar, North Queen Street, Belfast. I was 'living in' at the time and, with other student nurses, was wakened after midnight and asked to go to theatre recovery. My duty was to 'special' (one-to-one nursing) a male civilian who incurred terrible injuries from which, sadly, he did not recover. This man and his injuries are indelibly etched on my mind.

During the remainder of my time at the Royal most of my career as a post-registration student and a staff nurse was spent in medical wards and generally away from direct contact with casualties. The Troubles were never far away, however. For example, I experienced something of the effects of CS gas, albeit in a dilute form, as it wafted its way from an altercation in Dunville Park to the vicinity of the hospital's Grosvenor Road entrance where a couple of us hardy male off-duty student nurses had assembled to observe events!

Getting into and out of the hospital site was often problematical. I recall one night in particular when there had been a prison escape. All the street lights on the Grosvenor Road had been shot out. I drove at considerable speed in the eerie darkness ignoring the traffic lights, which were still working. On arrival at the hospital entrance

I found the gate had been closed early. A security officer with whom I had a good relationship let me in.

Searching the ward for bombs following hoax anonymous telephone calls was a task not described in the training curriculum. I recall doing this on perhaps two occasions under the guise of a 'quick tidy of the lockers' so as not to alarm the patients.

Violence and mental health

In June of 1972 I returned to live in Omagh and work at the Tyrone and Fermanagh Psychiatric Hospital as a staff nurse. Violence continued to escalate in the province. It did not, in my view, affect mental health inpatient services to the extent that one might have expected at that time. I was soon allocated for a three-year period to the community psychiatric nurse department – a burgeoning service in those days. It was in this role that one could detect the upcoming need for a new and more extensive and specialised kind of clinical services for stress and post-traumatic stress-related problems.

On a personal level I have many recollections of working in the community. One stands out in my mind, however. On my first day I rounded a corner on a quiet road on the Fermanagh/Monaghan border to be confronted with a large armoured army vehicle with its back doors open and soldiers diving into the drains and hedgerows. Stopping in a casual manner beside the first prostrate soldier, I was informed that there had been an exchange of small arms fire. Until that moment I had no idea how fast a car would travel in reverse gear!

The Omagh bombing

Tragedies and suffering continued to occur in Northern Ireland, England and the Republic of Ireland. Each morning's news bulletins brought more stories of atrocities and killings. In the thinking of many these were usually happening 'somewhere else'. For any Omagh residents with this mindset all was to change on the pleasant summer Saturday afternoon of 15 August 1998.

I was at home when the bomb exploded. Our daughter Grace, who was 12 years old at the time, was in town. A neighbour and I rushed into the town to try to find her, but we were immediately confronted with the extent of the devastation. Initially we could not find her, but as emergency services had arrived we decided to return in the hope that she had managed to get home. At the end of that agonising half-mile journey I was relieved beyond measure to see our daughter in the distance safe and well. She had met one of her teachers who had given her a lift home.

I ran the 200 metres or so to Tyrone County Hospital to see what I might be able to do. No training in surgical procedures, no tuition in wound care, no amount of lectures on psychology, no stories around the fireside of times gone by could prepare me for what was unfolding.

By this time most of the people still alive had been brought in. I have a vivid recollection of injured patients lying in the corridors. After reporting to the senior nurse I linked up by telephone with one of my managers in Tyrone & Fermanagh Hospital to confirm that all available personnel from there were needed, along with linen and all basic requirements that a situation like this demanded. I aligned myself with a badly injured lady who had been brought in on a door used as a makeshift stretcher. When she was taken to theatre I found myself in one of the wards where I spent most of the remainder of the day.

In a small rural community where many are known to one another it was heartbreaking to witness a father searching for his daughter, a mother collapsing when she saw the extent of her daughter's injuries for the first time, and others coming to terms with the reality that their loved one had not survived. Some of the memories of that dreadful day have become occluded in my mind. Perhaps that is my coping mechanism. Other memories remain vivid. For example, how sticky blood can be underfoot, the blood-soaked overalls of the duty maintenance officer acting in a role that I am sure he never had envisaged, the helicopters queuing in the sky as they waited to land to transfer patients to other hospitals for treatment.

At the end of a long and difficult day I walked the short distance back home. It was only then that I learned that our daughter Grace had been within 20 metres of the bomb when it exploded. Miraculously she escaped with only temporary hearing damage. For other families, many of whom were known to us, the outcome was so different.

In my childhood days, like everyone else in the community, I could not have envisaged what was to come in the course of my lifetime. I retired on August 9 2004, not only having observed the most profound changes in the profession of nursing in a generation, but having had direct personal experience of many traumatic Troubles-related events, including murder and attempted murder.

Even the quiet village of Pettigo, the place of my birth, was by no means immune to tragedy and grief.**"**

Violence erupts –
Bombs, booby traps and bullets
1969-1979

"Ulster nurses are shrugging off the headache imposed by the province's Troubles and soldiering on. I would say the Troubles are putting additional pressure on nurses because they have to provide a 24-hour service and in many circumstances they are the only people available to assist at a given moment in time."

Miss R Calvert, 1976
Secretary to Northern Ireland Board RCN

Rioting at Free Derry Corner, 1969

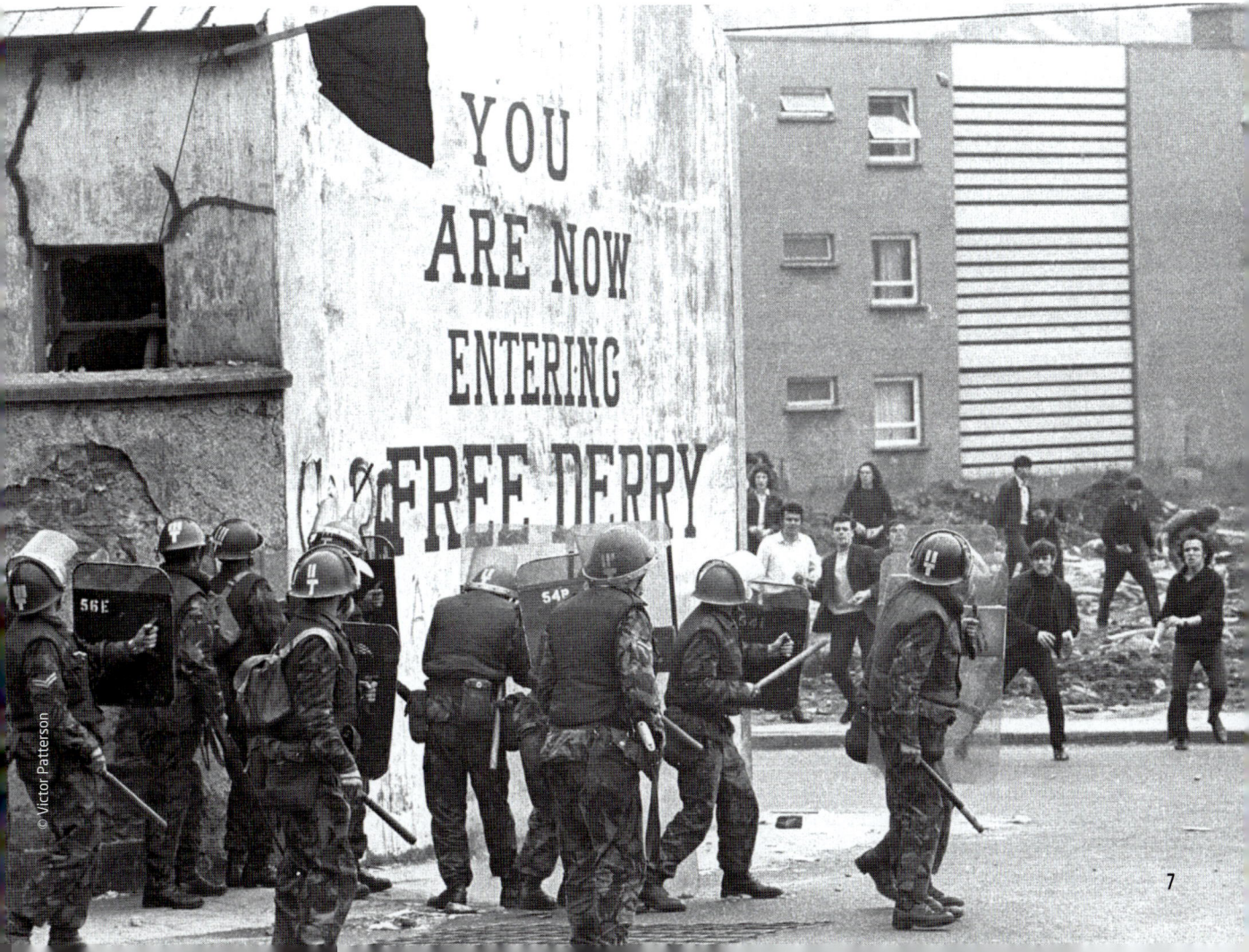

© Victor Patterson

1969-1979
Deaths 2,112
Injured 22,543[1][2]

August 1969 saw prolonged outbreaks of rioting in Derry/Londonderry, Belfast and to a lesser degree other provincial towns. The violence that erupted in Derry/Londonderry on 12 August 1969 escalated and lasted for three days. Meanwhile on 14-15 August houses in Bombay Street, West Belfast were burned. Tension was rising across Northern Ireland, civil disorder escalated and British troops were deployed onto the streets.

The violence of that weekend resulted in deaths and many hundreds of injuries. The riots also caused family displacement along adjoining Catholic and Protestant streets in Belfast, with many families moving from their homes in the North and West of the city. This unrest had a direct impact on health services. Following this weekend, violence escalated further. The army's presence did not bring peace and nurses began for the first time to see horrendous injuries from the impact of the unrest on local communities. The stories that follow are recollections from nurses who worked in Belfast and Derry/Londonderry at this time.

[1]Sutton M (2002) Appendix Statistical Summary. Annual Killings by Military and Paramilitary Groups (1969-2001). http://cain.ulst.ac.uk/sutton/book/index.html#append [February 20 2013.]

[2]Melaugh M, McKenna F, Brendan L (2003) Table NI-SEC-05: Persons Injured (number) due to the security situation in Northern Ireland (only), 1969 to 2003. CAIN Web Service. http://cain.ulst.ac.uk.ni/security.htm#05 [February 20 2013] And for all subsequent death/injured references.

Adapting to changing conditions

A night sister later reminisced...

"When civil disturbances began in 1969 it seemed that the hospital role changed from that of peaceful work to war-time work...

On the first night of severe riots 40 people were admitted, most having to have operations, and theatre staff worked non-stop for 48 hours. Casualty department seemed one mass of people – some injured, some visitors looking for relatives, all distraught and many not very polite.

During this very distressing time, sisters and nurses often stayed on duty all day and until late at night, and the students who had just started on the wards often came back at 8.30pm and stayed until midnight, in spite of gunfire and bombing in the area. These conditions made it difficult to get to the hospital, as there was no public transport, and walking along dark streets and hearing guns and bombs was, to say the least, an unpleasant experience. Many times it was safer, and more certain, just to stay in the hospital and not to try to go home.[3]**"**

[3]Royal Victoria Hospital League of Nurses magazine (1980) No.31, May.

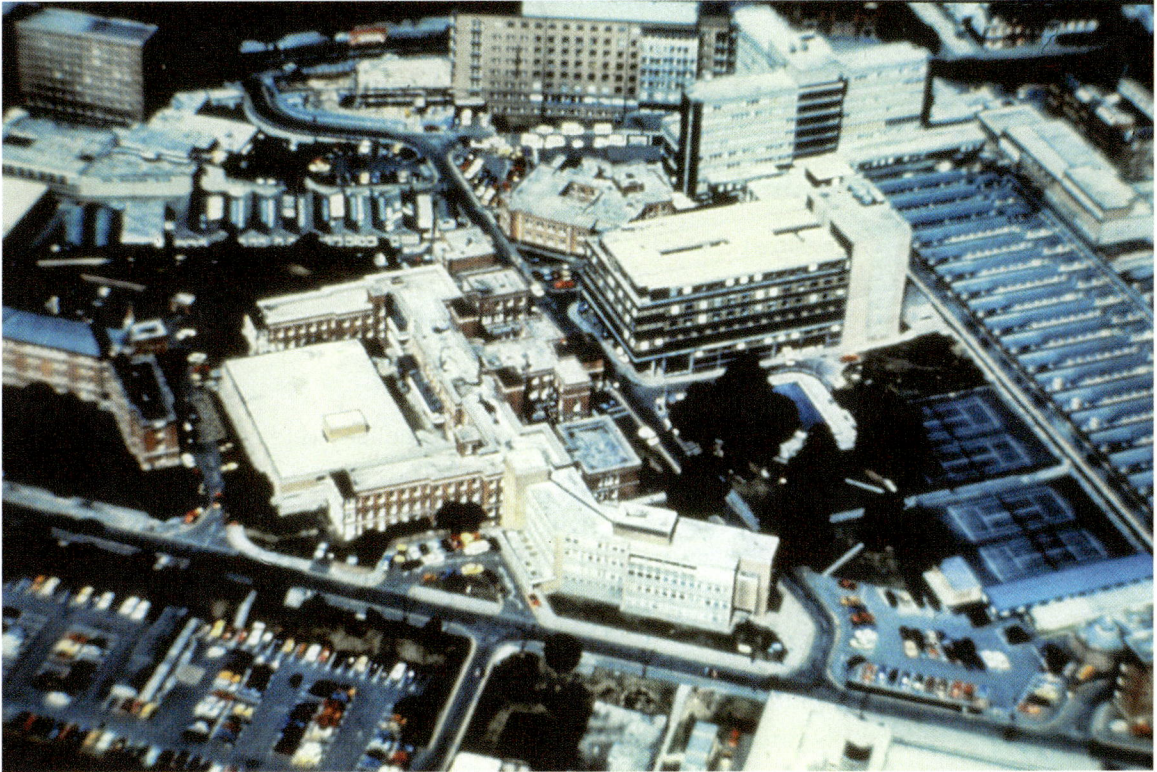
Royal Victoria Hospital

In Belfast, the Royal Victoria Hospital was at the centre of the disruption, flanked on all sides by streets that were directly affected by rioting, burning and gunfire.

A night of memories
14-15 August 1969

"Admissions on that night were 44, of these, 26 required surgery."
Theatre Sister

On the night of 14 August a theatre sister was contacted to return to work and open additional theatres for casualties being admitted. She recalls: "I saw bullet wounds for the first time." Not only was there concern about how to treat these effectively to ensure healing, but nursing and medical staff were faced with additional professional and ethical issues of dealing with forensic evidence. All bullets removed had to be labelled and retained. Some theatre nurses recalled the stress of being subpoenaed to give evidence in court about excised bullets and asked to account for missing information regarding the clothes of a victim.

"Subpoena that woman and bring the missing page of the clothing book to me on Monday!"
Belfast Barrister

In the absence of training or guidance on the management of such untoward events, one can only imagine the anxiety of working in a scenario where the first priority is to maintain and preserve life.

"At first we stitched up the bullet wounds, but then realised that this was not the best treatment. These wounds were subsequently managed by delayed primary closure."
Theatre Nurse

❝As a theatre sister in the Royal Victoria Hospital (RVH), Belfast, this was my introduction to dealing with patients injured as a result of the Troubles. In the days preceding the night of Thursday 14-15 August it was evident that a level of civil unrest was present in parts of the city. But the sudden escalation of violence, between 12 midnight and 3am, was unexpected and unprecedented.

Rioting in the narrow streets surrounding the hospital resulted in a number of injured being admitted, some with gunshot wounds. The hospital was surrounded with barricades and fires, isolated within the zone of rioting. Access was difficult and dangerous.

Just before midnight a colleague and I were contacted and asked to return to duty to open additional theatres. Although I lived in a high-rise block of flats near the hospital and was able to observe some of the activity in surrounding areas, I did not realise the extent of the disturbances as we walked across the hospital grounds. I remember having to fall to the ground in response to someone shouting at us to do so. Later, we were told that a gunman was thought to be in the grounds.

Three operating rooms worked continuously throughout the night. Most of the gunshot wounds were to limbs. Metal foreign bodies,

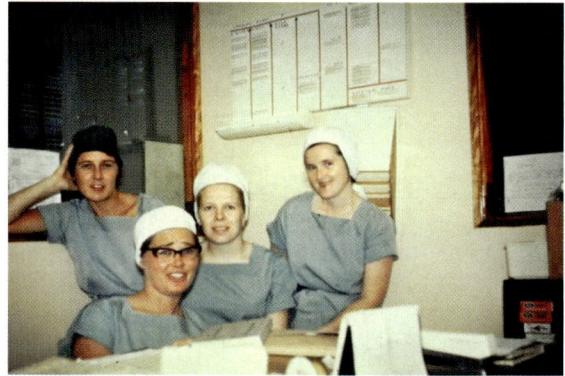
Theatre Nurses 1970

bullets and pellets were among the objects removed. These had to be accurately labelled, safely stored and later handed over to the authorities.

As morning approached and a considerable workload still remained, a decision was taken to cancel elective surgery that Friday. I remember contacting medical staff in the early morning hours to advise them of this decision. All were disbelieving when they answered the phone.

Although not having dealt with gunshot wounds before, it was the surrounding political and legal issues and the background against which these injuries occurred that gave concern that night.

Isolated within the zone of rioting and with limited communication with outside events, we worked on. Had the situation peaked? Was it contained locally or was it spreading province-wide? Those on duty were also feeling concerned for family and friends. There was a feeling that it was all 'unreal'. Was this really happening? Looking back I had no concept then, that in the next 20-plus years, I would be involved in many more incidents. They were often major bomb blasts, with greater numbers of casualties resulting in deaths and severe injuries.

For anyone reading this more than 40 years later, it may be difficult to appreciate why I remember that night in particular. Things were different then. Emergencies to me meant perforated appendix or trauma from a car accident. Hospital disaster plans were more basic. Now they reflect the experience gained from managing the many disasters and atrocities which have happened worldwide in the years since 1969.

Communications were more limited with no mobile phones and other such technologies. Sterile goods were sterilised on-site, not pre-packed. There were limited disposable items. This meant more time preparing sterile trolleys. Counselling services did not exist. New surgical technologies have developed as a result of trauma treated over many years. Things that remain the same are the effects on patients, staff, their families, friends and colleagues.❞

Scrub or runner?

A staff nurse thought it was going to be a quiet night, but she was mistaken...

❛❛When I went on night duty as Staff Nurse in charge of theatres on Thursday 14 August, I was told there were two theatres set up ready for use and that some members of staff would be phoning about midnight to see if all was 'quiet'. I said I didn't think anything was going to happen. How wrong I was!

In fact when staff phoned in, all was quiet, but not for long. A short time later I received a call from Night Sister telling me there were two patients coming to theatre. I asked her: 'What for?' She replied: 'One in the abdomen and one in the thigh.' 'One what?' I asked her. 'Gunshot wounds' was her response. I had no idea they had started shooting outside the hospital.

Fortunately one of the sisters who lived nearby knew what was happening and arrived very soon, followed by many other staff. Sister took charge and directed staff to go to a theatre and either 'scrub' or be a 'runner'. The rest of the night all theatres were working and, as the day staff came on duty, the night staff were able to go home. We were the lucky ones as many of the staff coming on duty on Friday were there for most of the weekend.❞

"Keep looking positive!"

A sister in the "take-in" ward at the Royal Victoria Hospital (RVH) has a vivid memory of 15 August 1969. At that time the major Belfast hospitals were on a rota for admitting medical and surgical emergency admissions. Ambulances took casualties to accident and emergency departments according to the rota. The on-call hospital had to ensure that they had empty beds for "take-in".

❛❛That day I was the junior (teaching) sister on duty in surgical wards 11-12 at the RVH, with Professor Harold Rodgers as the consultant. There had been reports of trouble in Londonderry leading up to this date, but I did not think that was going to affect me. However, rioting and shootings erupted on the streets of West Belfast that day.

All day and evening, patients were pushed in on trolleys to our ward. We were on 'Take-in'. The patients mostly had gunshot wounds. It was so hectic and so surreal.

We were told we could not leave the hospital for our safety so I spent the night with others in the west wing. We looked out the windows and could see flames and smoke billowing into the night air where factories had been set on fire on the Falls Road. I felt great sadness to see such a sight.

I will always remember the following morning when Professor Rodgers did his ward round. He was in a pristine white coat with a rose in his lapel. I enquired politely whether he was going somewhere special. He replied it was most important that morale must be kept up and to look positive in the midst of such trauma.

Another memory at a later date is the 11-year-old girl who had been having symptoms of appendicitis at home but her parents were too scared to bring her through the rioting. When they eventually brought her the appendix had perforated and she was very ill. She subsequently developed a pelvic abscess. Happily, after many weeks she was well enough to go home.**"**

A lost friend

"I was a theatre sister in the Royal Victoria Hospital when the conflict started. I remember being the scrub nurse for a soldier who had sustained a gunshot wound to the head and was bleeding profusely.

We could not save him. At that time, if the casualty was a soldier, the army provided the security outside the theatre. I was quite emotional as I dressed his wounds and left the theatre to compose myself. I came face to face with the soldier who was the guard. 'That didn't take long. Is he going to be alright? He's my best friend,' he said. I replied: 'The surgeon will speak to you.' He only looked about 18 years of age.**"**

Midwife on the periphery

"In 1969, I was a Midwifery Sister on night duty in the labour ward in the Royal Maternity Hospital (RMH), Belfast, now known as the Royal Jubilee Maternity Hospital, situated close to the Royal Victoria Hospital (RVH). The labour ward at that time directly faced the RVH.

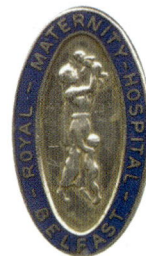

Because of the location, labour ward staff quickly became aware of the developing social unrest in the city. There was a great increase in ambulance and police activity going to the A&E department. We quickly became familiar with the sounds of gunfire, bombs, followed by the sirens and police cars as they sped to the A&E unit.

Friday 15 August saw an event that transformed the 'social unrest' into what came to be called the Troubles and influenced the next 30 years. On that Friday there were just 20 liveable houses left in the street after a Loyalist gang attacked and burned the other 45 Catholic houses. Many families were left homeless. It was a great recruitment opportunity for the IRA. For the first time later that day soldiers were seen on the streets of Belfast. The first night that blast bombs were thrown, I stopped counting after 30.

Midwifery staff found themselves in a new role in dealing with the social aftermath of various incidents including the Lower Falls fire. They had to cope with the traumatised mothers' grief, not so much for the ruined furniture and so on, as for the loss of family photographs and memorabilia of their children's early years. Life became increasingly difficult for community midwives doing their rounds, and for mothers in labour needing to travel to the RMH. That eventually led to a change in the management of these mothers.

Another seminal event was the introduction of Internment on 9 August 1971 by the British government, when 342 men were arrested without trial in 'Operation Demetrius'. The banging of dustbin lids by women and children as a warning that security forces were in the area became an annual feature every 9th of August after that. Over 7,000 fled their homes and became displaced people, taking refuge in schools and church halls. Of this number, around 2,500 people fled to the Republic of Ireland. There were 24 deaths.

As we welcomed yet another beautiful baby, we pondered on what sort of a world they would grow up in.

In the early 1970s, a new labour suite opened on the opposite side of the RMH, so that with double-glazing the staff did not hear the events of the outer world so easily. But an incident one night could have had devastating consequences.

There was a very large plate glass window in the waiting room of the new building. This particular night a number of us were enjoying a well-earned cup of tea, sitting directly opposite this window, when a bomb went off close by. We watched in horror as this window started to cave in before our eyes but thankfully returned to its position again. It was one of those situations one had to experience to believe. The casualty rate would have been high with possible fatalities if the window had shattered.

On a lighter note, coming off night duty years later, helicopters with searchlights had become a nightly feature where I lived. Needless to say sleep was interrupted due to the continuous drone

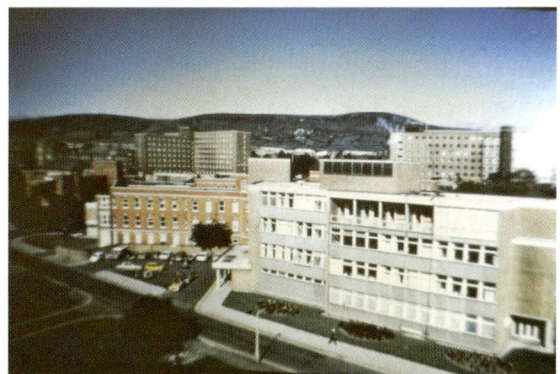

The Royal Maternity Hospital, now the Royal Jubilee

and the bright light. One weekend, my husband and I decided to get away to get a good night's sleep. We travelled to my parents' home in Co Tyrone. Imagine our chagrin when on arrival the first thing we saw was six helicopters parked in the field behind the house. We could only laugh!**"**

Nursing pride

Miss Mary Kathleen Robb was Matron of the Royal Victoria Hospital (RVH) Belfast from 1966 to 1973 and District Administrative Nursing Officer from 1973 (when she was awarded an OBE) until her retirement in 1984. A loyal and involved member of the Royal College of Nursing, she was made a Fellow in 1977 and presented with a lifetime achievement award in 2003. She has many memories of working through the Troubles.

"I had a tremendous pride in the staff throughout the Troubles."
Miss Robb's Matron's Report, 1969

"Northern Ireland was 'headline news' many times in 1969, and during the late summer and autumn months our hospital was surrounded by fighting, fires and people who, through fear, had encamped themselves behind man-made barricades.

During this time the 'Royal' team spirit was never stronger, extending from senior consultants and administrators down to the porters, whose sudden presence in the late evening usually heralded unrest outside. Overnight the west wing became a hotel, and never before in its history did it house such a variety of personnel, including senior consultant staff. The sisters all undertook extra duties, and this included our colleagues from the School of Nursing who joined us after school hours to ensure that there was always a strong senior nursing team available at night. The student nurses came to our office daily to offer their help, and deserve special mention, as do the medical students who gave long hours of service both outside as well as within the hospital.

The hospital service reserve were prepared to tackle any task, even acting as taxi drivers when patients were being moved to outside hospitals to ensure that sufficient beds would be available for casualties. Many phone calls were received from the public offering help, including ex-RVH nurses.

During this period the admission of patients on the waiting list for surgery decreased, resulting in a busy aftermath. Then the winter influenza epidemic struck, and to cope with the sharp increase in medical admissions, the cardiothoracic, gynaecological, eye, ear, nose and throat, dermatology and metabolic wards were all used in rotation as medical wards. Again staff volunteered for extra duties to cope with the increased workload and replace the many nurses who were off sick. Medical students undertook nursing duties and at the peak of the epidemic, health visitors were seconded and proved to be invaluable, acting as a wonderful stimulus to the allocation office, which had the unenviable task of trying to provide 24-hour nursing cover to all wards and departments.[4]**"**

[4] Royal Victoria Hospital League of Nurses magazine (1970) M. Kathleen Robb

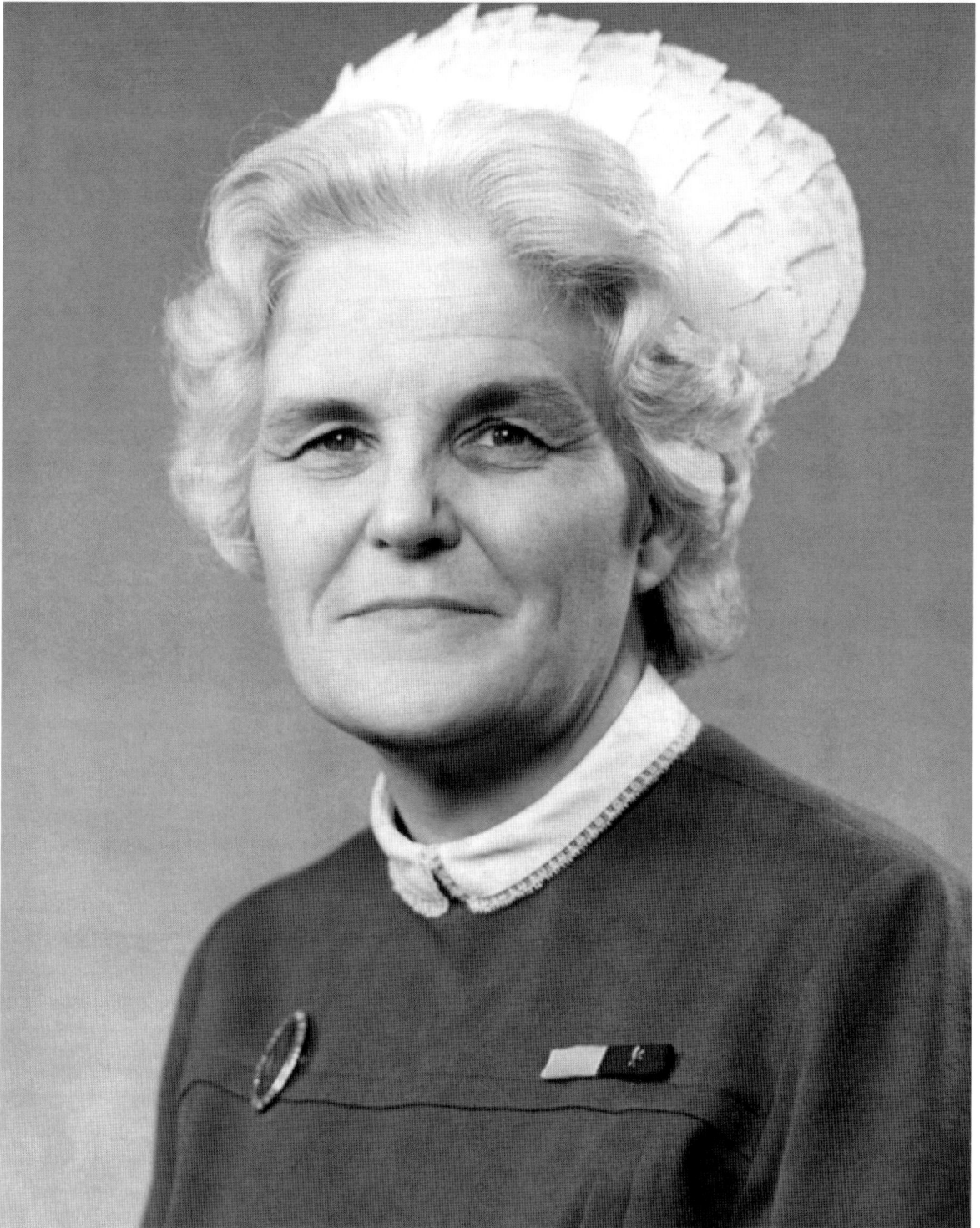

Miss Robb, Matron RVH: "We were surrounded by fighting and fires … but team spirit was never stronger."

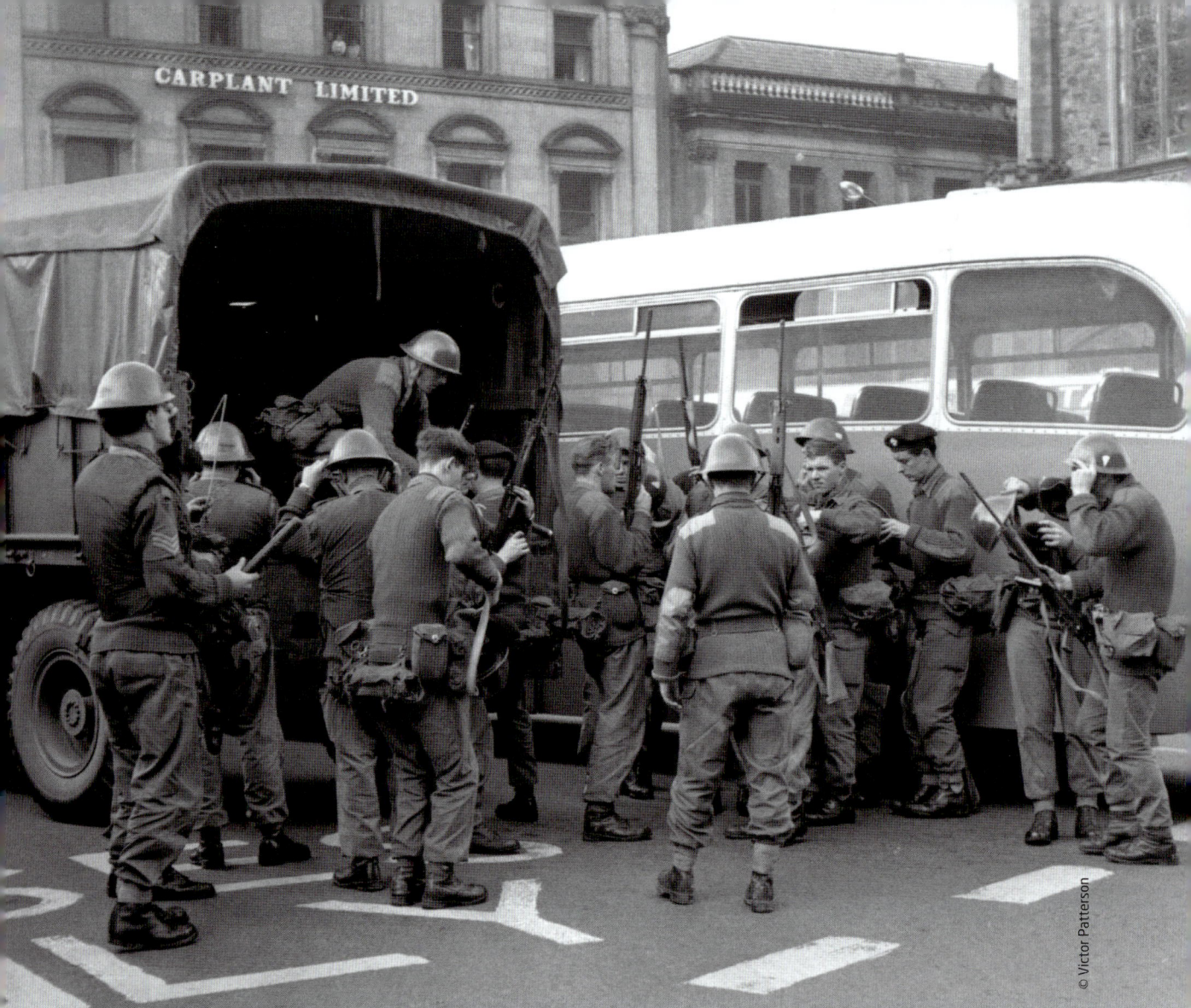

© Victor Patterson

Troops arrive in Derry/Londonderry, 1969

Bombs in Derry

While nurses in Belfast were seeing casualties of rioting and civil disorder for the first time, so too were nurses in Altnagelvin Hospital, Derry/Londonderry. Throughout 1969 there were frequent skirmishes between civil rights movement marchers and police. On 12 August rioting erupted following the annual Apprentice Boys march and lasted for three days until the arrival of the British army on 14 August at the request of the Stormont government. Derry/Londonderry, being a much smaller city than Belfast, it was a community in which nearly everyone knew everyone. Nurses working in the hospital talked of their fear and concern that they would know or be related to casualties admitted. Staff remember having to cope with emergency admissions into the accident and emergency unit with only a

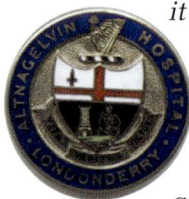

student workforce to rely on. Nurses also recalled the support provided by ancillary staff who assisted in so many ways, including making cups of tea for distressed non-injured casualties and their relatives.

The following stories are from nurses working in Altnagelvin Hospital...

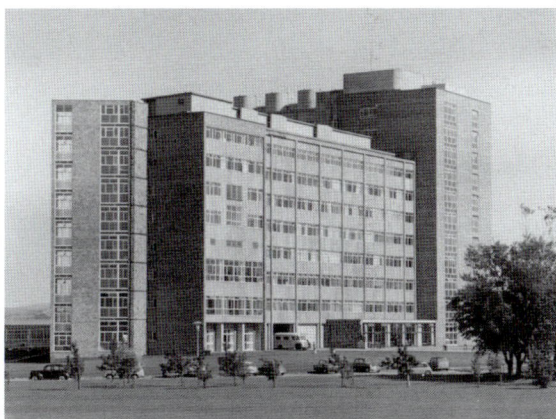

Altnagelvin Hospital circa 1969

The lost glasses

❝That afternoon in A&E I was one of three student nurses on duty, and I was carrying the drugs keys. In those years, there were afternoons when there was no trained staff to cover A&E.

Luckily, that afternoon I had no surgery day cases. The message came through that three bombs had exploded in the city. We had no experience of how to cope. It was all new to us. The doctor on duty worked three afternoons a week. Her husband was a clergyman newly arrived in Donegal, and she was in her fifties and had decided to return to medicine.

First through the door came a boy who had been 'tarred and feathered', accompanied by two pals. I put them in a room and gave them some towels and a tin of Swarfega and told them to get on with it.

Then the casualty doors opened and my knees went weak... but I soon recovered. We received 16 casualties and a lot of hysterical people. Fortunately none of the latter was too badly injured. I put them into the casualty wards, which had eight beds, and the kitchen ladies made them tea and toast and got them settled. When they had calmed, we then discharged them home by ambulance.

Some of the casualties needed X-rays and some had to be sutured. But we got through it all, despite our lack of experience. We simply used common sense, our good training and co-operation with each other. Four patients were admitted to A&E, including a mother and daughter from Buncrana. One of the buildings blown up was Etam's, a lingerie store. The manager was visiting from London. He had lost his glasses, so I contacted a lady in the X-ray department whose boyfriend was an optician with a view to arranging a replacement set. But in the meantime his own glasses were found and returned to him. Personnel from head office in London called the hospital to enquire about their store manager and I put him on the line so that they could receive first-hand assurance that he was not seriously injured.

When hand-over came at 5pm, normality had been restored in the department.

That was my first experience of nursing during the Troubles. It was certainly a steep learning curve and from then on we were always improving. And of course we had many worse days after that."

An angel in the kitchen

Another staff nurse recalls...

"One horrific night in casualty in the late 1970s, I was on duty with a student nurse. As well as dealing with casualties, we had to look after an eight-bed admission ward.

It started with several patients coming in with gunshot wounds. Then there was an explosion across the city. Help arrived from everywhere in the hospital and everyone from doctors and nurses to radiographers, ambulance crews and porters weighed in and lent a hand. Senior staff rolled up their sleeves, washed bloody floors and did anything that was necessary. We were eventually getting cleared up around 5am, when we had a report of another explosion and within minutes our department was full again.

It was a hectic night, so, when the day staff arrived, we went into the kitchen for our first tea and toast of the shift. There the 'post-mortem' started as we discussed what had happened, what everyone had seen and done. Ambulance crew, doctors, nurses, porters and radiographers were all there. We discussed everything we did that night and what, if anything, we could have done better. We also talked about how we felt.

Everyone had a story and a worry about what had happened.

From the middle of the crowded kitchen a voice said: 'Well dears, did you do your best?' We looked around, and there stood one of our domestics, a small lady who had been making us tea and listening in to our conversations. After a few moments thought, I said 'Yes' and the others agreed. We had done the best we could and so we could go home to bed content with that reassurance.

This was our counselling."

Just a normal night duty?

"Sunday 15 August 1971 was a very eventful day in my life."

"I had started nursing in September 1969 at Altnagelvin Hospital; before that I had been a member of the Order of Malta carrying out the normal first-aid duties associated with the organisation. The Troubles changed all that as I found myself administering first aid in the Bogside from day one of the Battle of the Bogside. Most days I left after work to take up duty in one of the various first-aid posts which we opened as needs prevailed. During August 1971 we were using St Mary's Girls School in the Creggan estate.

I was on duty there as the nurse in charge on that eventful night.

An off-duty Catholic policeman, who was home visiting his family in the Bogside, was recognised and attacked by a crowd, a short distance from St Eugene's Cathedral. Word got through to the cathedral and Father Daly and Father O'Neill came to his rescue. The large crowd refused to let him be taken to hospital, but after another priest arrived, they were allowed to bring him to our first-aid post.

I received word of his imminent arrival and was given instructions to move the families who were using the school as a refuge to the upper floors of the building. When he arrived, he was in a lot of pain, distressed and very frightened, so we laid him on a stretcher and treated his injuries.

Meanwhile the crowd, which had followed the car to the Creggan, had started to increase in size and was demanding that the police officer be handed over to them immediately. Tensions were running high but we were determined that our patient would only leave us to go to hospital.

A short time later a local GP, Dr McCabe, arrived and began contacting someone by phone in Stormont. I heard a commotion in the corridor and to my shock I saw three armed and masked men stating they were members of a Provisional IRA unit. Realising we were in a well-lit room, we moved our patient to a small store room. Unfortunately it was also well lit with large windows. We could not see out but those outside could see in, so we stayed low to the floor.

Some months later I was told that there were individuals trying to get a shot at the policeman, but I was blocking their view and, because they respected the neutrality of our Knights of Malta organisation, they did not take a shot for fear of shooting me.

A short time later we were informed that the masked men wanted to see our patient. We were terrified of course, but we were not given a choice so they were given access to see him. They asked me what I thought of his condition and I insisted that he needed hospital admission. Eventually they left and we were told that negotiations were taking place between the British army and the RUC (who were running the Border checkpoints with the army), the Stormont authorities and the Southern government.

Journey to Letterkenny Hospital
The next thing I remember is that the decision was made to move our patient, by ambulance, to Letterkenny Hospital across the border in Donegal. I was to go as a nurse with a doctor and a priest, but just as we were about to move off, another man, a stranger to us, boarded the ambulance. He seemed to have been involved in the negotiating.

We were stopped at the Letterkenny Road checkpoint close to the border, even though we were supposed to be allowed safe passage. The unknown man, who never gave his name, got out of the ambulance and spoke to the army and the RUC. A short time later he came back and told us to drive on.

As we drove in pitch darkness, a car came towards us from Letterkenny, stopped in the middle of the road, turned and tried to overtake us. Someone in the ambulance said: 'It must be the IRA.' At this I was really frightened, but our unknown friend reassured us that all was okay. Taking no chances the driver drove at speed so we couldn't be overtaken.

It was only when we reached the lights of the Letterkenny Hospital that we realised the car had contained a plain-clothes Garda team there to escort us safely on our journey. All I could see were bright lights, cameras and armed Irish army personnel, guarding the ambulance. My thoughts at that time were that if my mother knew what happened, I would have been in real trouble, as she assumed I spent my nights in the nurses' home. I couldn't be caught on camera, so I threw a blanket over myself and our patient and we quickly made our way inside.

I settled and reassured the policeman in case he was worried about being left alone there without knowing what was going to happen. When I left him to get some tea, our unknown friend went in to speak to him. As we were about to leave for home, I called in to speak to the patient and he seemed more relaxed and not as worried as before.

Journey back home

On the way home, as we approached the Letterkenny Road checkpoint, things didn't feel right. We were stopped again by some angry security personnel, so our unknown friend went out to speak to them. I remember looking out of the window and seeing the RUC remonstrating with the British army.

Our 'friend' ran back to the ambulance telling everyone to get on the floor and to drive as fast as we could. We all huddled together on the floor saying our prayers as the ambulance reached speeds I didn't think it could do.

We only relaxed when we approached Derry. Our unknown friend asked to be left off at his hotel where we were met by a large group of anxious people. We understood their anxiety when they told us they had monitored radio transmissions from the border and, because they had heard threats to kill us, assumed we were all dead.

We left the City Hotel and took Father Daly home to the cathedral and I went back to the first-aid post intending to get some sleep but, due to casualties resulting from British army raids, I had none at all. Around about 6am, I walked from the first-aid post to the Guildhall where I caught the early bus to Altnagelvin Hospital, arriving in time to begin my normal day's duty.

Six months later, Father (later Bishop) Daly was invited to visit the US Congress in Washington DC. I remember him telling me that he was approached by a man who asked did he not remember him. Bishop Daly couldn't until he said: 'Do you not remember that fateful night when we were nearly shot dead at the Letterkenny Road checkpoint?'

Bishop Daly later wrote in his book 'Mister, Are You A Priest?' about our unknown man: 'I do not know to this day what his precise role was in Creggan on that night. He was one of several mysterious and sinister people from various parts of the world who circulated in Derry during those years.'[5] **"**

---

[5]Edward Daly (2000) *Mister, Are You A Priest?* Four Courts Press, Dublin.

In later years

"In 1979 I was a ward sister in a medical ward at the Royal Victoria Hospital. One morning I arrived on duty and as usual walked around each patient to see how they were.

Unbeknownst to me a patient had been admitted overnight directly to the ward and was screened from view of the other patients. I was caught off guard, totally overcome with shock at the sight of the person sitting up looking at me.

The patient had multiple amputations and various sensory impairments. The artificial limbs were lying beside the bed. This young adult had been a victim of an explosion seven years earlier.

I often worry if my face that morning betrayed my horror of those injuries. I was angry at such needless pain and anguish caused to a young life and often wonder how many other people have been similarly physically and psychologically damaged, living a life so different to that of their adolescent dreams."

Community nursing
in 1969 and early 1970s

❝When the shooting started outside the clinic we just got under our desks and continued completing our records.❞

School Nurse

Soldiers on duty in the Crumlin Road area of Belfast, 1971

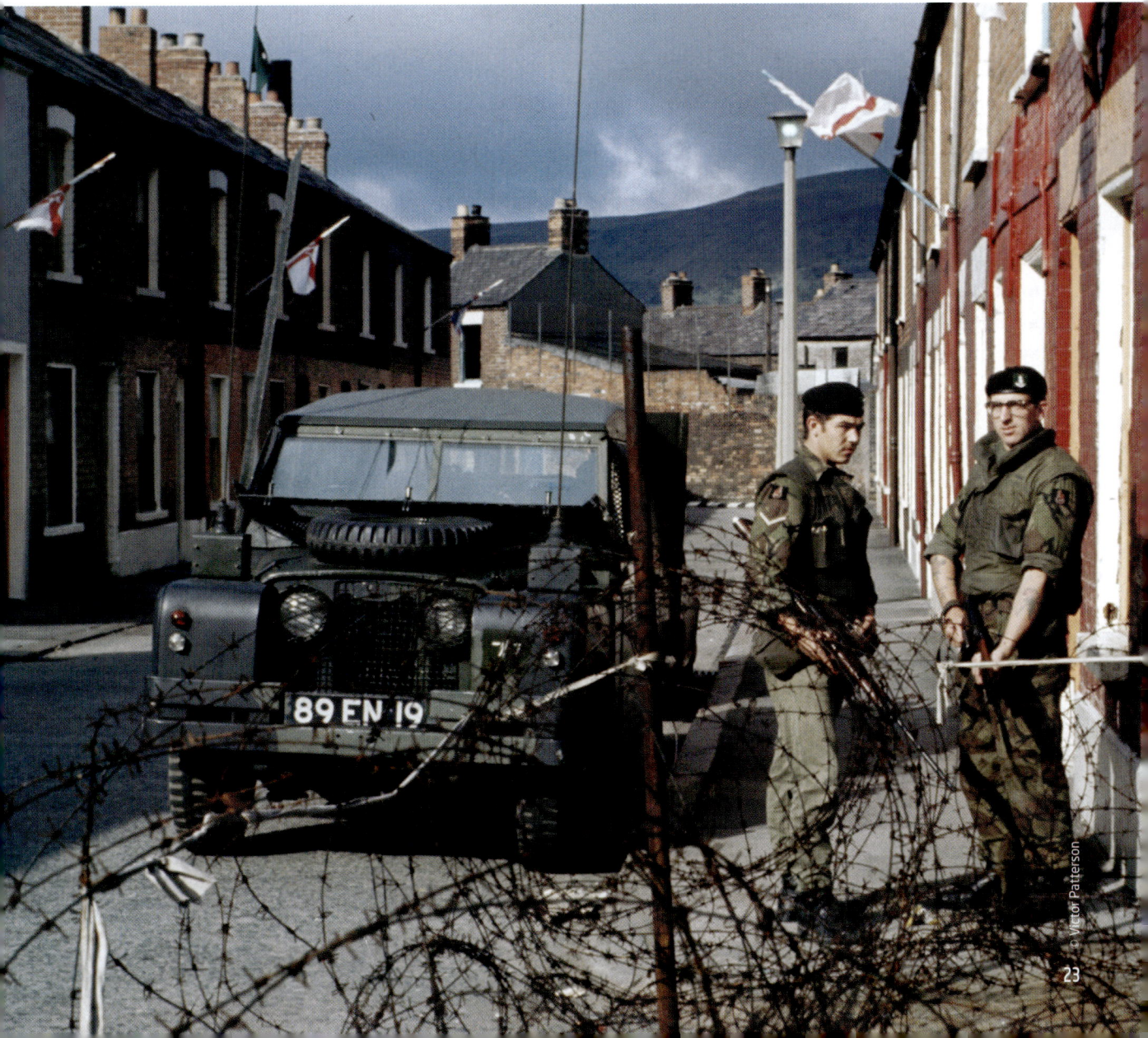

© Victor Patterson

When violent civil unrest broke out in 1969, community nurses were still employed by City Corporations or County Councils. A health visitor recalls her newly qualified experiences.

Health visiting in a conflict area

"Too dangerous for my council workers to go up there nurse, the very bin men are being shot at."
Council Official

"About a year after qualifying as a health visitor in 1969 I was based with many other community nurses and our first line supervisors at Cupar Street Health Clinic on the lower Falls Road. An army look-out post was already in situ on what was considered neutral territory, our front doorstep. This most certainly would have made us a target for bombers and snipers though none of us ever questioned the wisdom of its presence.

My caseload was drawn mainly from the right-hand side of the Springfield Road and included all the post-war housing estates on that side. These were by now polarising into Catholic and Protestant enclaves, both hugely influenced by paramilitary organisations and activists. I experienced no problems on religious grounds, moving freely between the two communities, apparently accepted by 'both' as 'one of them'.

Sometimes I saw and heard things which it would have been better that I had not. My golden rule was that my role was health promotion among these people irrespective of their religion, politics or paramilitary activities. When you work closely in communities such as these it is amazing how quickly you begin to walk in their shoes and see things from their perspective and you have to earn their trust rather than having it as of right. Population movement through intimidation was widespread and keeping track of vulnerable families was not easy. Squatters would appear from nowhere sometimes to houses where the electric had been disconnected. A cold environment indeed for any small baby or toddler on a winter's day.

In addition to the run of problems associated with any conurbation there were many extra challenges thrown up by the conflict. Failure to keep antenatal, hospital or clinic appointments was commonplace. The excuses given were 'it's too dangerous to go down there nurse'; 'the buses might go off and I wouldn't get home again'. Bus services were often withdrawn at short notice during street violence.

This fear of travel out of people's safe zones was endemic and the consequent self-imposed isolation was an underlying factor in the increased depression rates, especially among young mothers with small children. Antidepressant use was widespread and people shared round their 'nerve tablets' with others during moments of crisis.

Environmental nuisances such as blocked rubbish chutes in the low-rise flats were common. Piles of rubbish accumulated to become rich breeding grounds for rats and flies. Phone calls produced responses such as 'too dangerous for my council workers to go up there nurse, the very bin men are being shot at'.

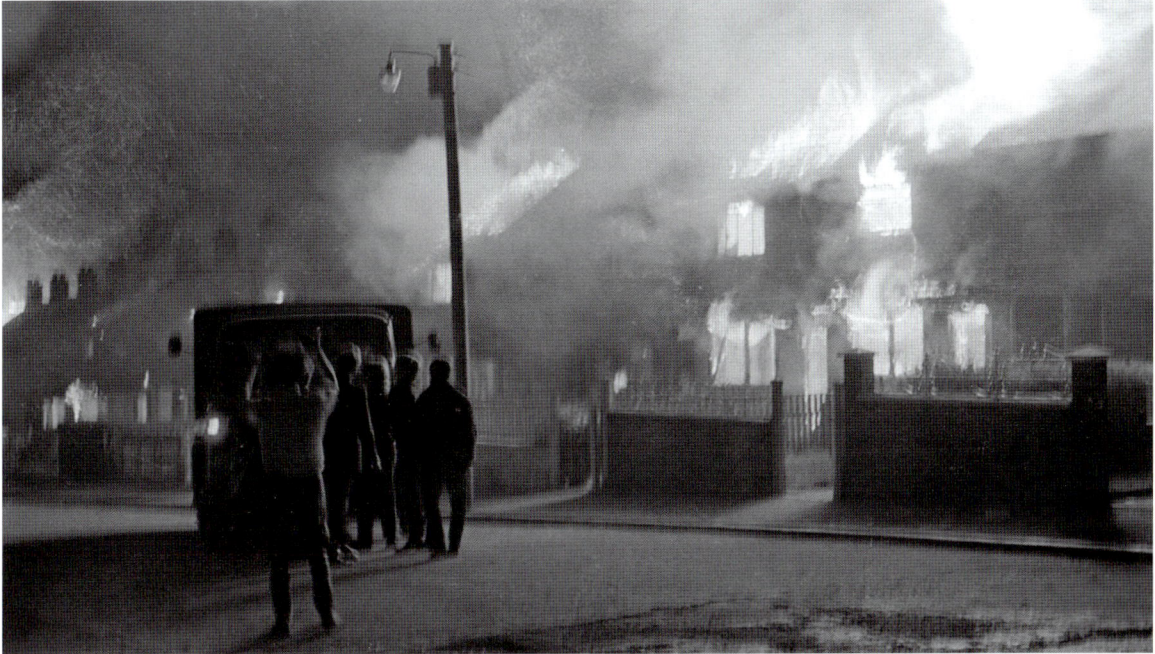

Post-internment rioting in North West Belfast, 1971

This indeed was a fact. All local government workers could be considered legitimate targets. Despite this I never felt personally threatened. To make sure my face was familiar, I frequently parked my car on the periphery of the estates and walked so that the people and also the security forces recognised me as a regular. It was important to acknowledge any paramilitaries manning barricades – 'I'm the community nurse on my way to such and such a street/park' usually got me through without problems. Sudden erection of illegal roadblocks could see any escape route made difficult, but usually one of your families could negotiate your safe exit. You also learned to read the signals of impending trouble; quiet streets, closed doors – it would have been foolish to remain in an area when the bin lids were being rattled – the local neighbourhood alarm system."

Reflections on a visit to elderly displaced pensioners in 1969

"Working in a conflict area meant routine duties had often to be shelved when other urgent problems cropped up. Following the destruction of a whole street during rioting on the Falls Road, a number of elderly residents were temporarily re-housed in caravans on rough waste ground further up the Falls Road. The Medical Officer requested a health and social needs review and report, and the task was delegated to me.

My immediate reaction was not enthusiastic. As a representative of the local government health team I was unsure what my reception would be, not to mention coping with the distress and perhaps hostility to be expected from people who had lost their entire home and possessions.

My fears were unfounded. These elderly citizens, all pensioners, could not believe that a 'welfare nurse' (their terminology for a health visitor) had been sent to check on them and offer assistance where possible. Their welcome was overwhelming and unanimous. All were grateful to have survived, alive and well, and have a roof, however temporary, over their heads. Yes, there were problems, such as lost pension books – social services had already an interim payment system set up; medications had to be sorted and re-established – 'I didn't get time in the confusion, nurse, to lift my heart tablets'.

There were many practical hazards. Three steep steps outside their doors to be negotiated without handrails for someone with stiff knees or a Zimmer are not conducive to safety. Most of the practical problems however had solutions or could be referred to other health team members. But when it came to more personal losses, apart from giving a listening ear, it was beyond me. 'My cat is still missing but I'm hopeful she will turn up somewhere yet'; 'All my photographs went up in smoke, even of my wedding day'.

The parting words of one of these redoubtable ladies stays with me: 'I was burned out in 1921, nurse, but I have had no bother 'til now. I got over it then and I will get over it this time too, God willing.' As I drove away full of admiration – and full of tea – for the sheer resilience of these retired citizens, mostly mill workers of yesteryear, I realised, perhaps for the first time in my life, just how invincible the human spirit is. "

The longest night

"Early in the 1970s in West Belfast, when the confrontation between the two communities was at its height, night emergency centres were established for families with small children left homeless by the Troubles or who were too frightened to spend the night in their own areas. As in the Blitz these reception centres were usually in schools or church halls or any building with a large enough floor space to accommodate mattresses, sleeping bags and so on.

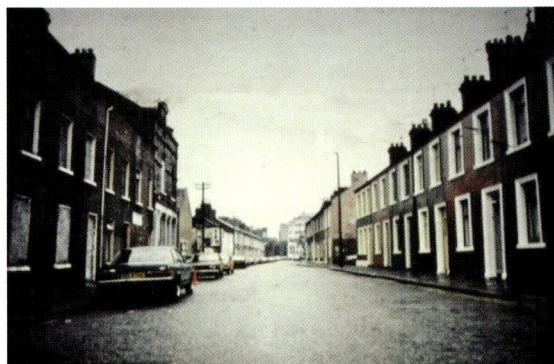

Belfast street near the Royal Victoria Hospital in the 1970s

The Chief Medical Officer for Belfast decreed that since groups were largely mothers with babies and young children, a qualified nurse must be present in a supervisory capacity, for example to oversee the preparation of infant feeds, minimising the risk of spread of infection.

On my first designated night I arrived between 8pm and 9pm at a large school hall on the Upper Falls Road. Already the place was crowded with mothers, babies and toddlers, all trying to claim a sleeping space on the floor of the gym. We had access to kitchen facilities with tea, coffee and infant feeding supplies available. Most people had brought sandwiches and biscuits for supper. If there was a telephone it was in the Head's office, which was locked, so we had no external means of communication.

There was no first-aid equipment of any kind and I had not had the wit or foresight to pre-empt this or I might have come prepared.

On checking my charges for the night I was most alarmed to find I had two very pregnant women, one almost full term, and two very stressed, asthmatic children among the group. When I discovered that outside on the Falls Road a barricade of burned-out vehicles was in the process of being erected between us and the Royal Group of Hospitals, I was even more dismayed.

I asked the paramilitaries present the whereabouts of the nearest telephone – no, they had no idea. I explained about the pregnant women and the sick children and the possibility of getting an ambulance in an emergency. Their reply was: 'No vehicle of any kind will get through here tonight – just do the best you can.'

Since midwifery was never my strong point and my only equipment was a pair of nail scissors, I was far from calm as I began to help the families bed down for the long night ahead. These people were tired, stressed and frightened, as indeed I was too, but for different reasons. I was also angry about having been put in this position without proper preparation or basic appropriate facilities.

It was a long night! Children coughed and wheezed and babies whimpered. The ventilation was poor and the air fetid with the smell of unwashed bodies, unchanged nappies and fear. Now and then a lighted cigarette glowed in the half light. I watched each one in case of an accidental fire as we had no emergency evacuation plans whatsoever.

As I did my supervisory night patrols I envied Florence Nightingale – at least she had a lamp and disinfectant! Outside the night was full of bangs and bumps, and raised voices and running footsteps round the building. Every so often the door opened and a strange male, obviously one of the paramilitaries, looked in, nodded and retreated without conversation.

Once a lad aged about 12-14 years rushed in, rummaged through a box of tissues on the table before me and retrieved a hidden knife. I tried to stop him, reasoning with him that he was too young to be involved in knife warfare. His reply was: 'If I have to defend myself and my mates I will use it if I have to.'

Morning came without further incident. I hoped my car would still be there to take me home. It was.

As soon as we returned to normal duty we held a meeting with our colleagues to discuss the impossible situations we had experienced. The more vocal amongst us were selected to take our grievances to our management at headquarters where we were met by the head of the medical and nursing management team of the day. Personally in the past I had always found our bosses helpful, approachable and willing to listen. They were less so on this occasion.

Our demands included:

- Free taxis to take us to and from the centres – this was refused on the grounds that our personal insurances covered us.
- First-aid equipment including 'dressing and midwifery packs' – this would be considered.
- Simple medications – refused as people were expected to bring their own supplies.
- Two nurses per night to each centre for professional and moral support – also refused on a staff shortage basis.
- We sought clarification of our roles and duties as health visitors, arguing that practical nursing and night duty were not within our remit hence we did not feel legally covered to do it.

On this point we were also defeated by the last clause of our contract which was set before us and which, as well as listing our health visiting duties, stated: 'Any other duties which the Medical Officer shall deem necessary from time to time.' The Medical Officer concerned was adamant he was acting within his powers and the best interests of those caught up in the emergency. We left the office feeling angry, dispirited and undervalued – our lives not even worth a taxi fare.

However, shortly afterwards a new policy came into force. All emergency night centres would thereafter be run by volunteer nurses from our teams. Many of my colleagues did volunteer. I was not one of them. The centres became unnecessary shortly after this as the security forces gained control over the street violence. For my part, working in a conflict area was challenging but never dull – frustrating at times but very rewarding.**"**

A street disappears

"Many memorable moments while health visiting in the troubled areas of Belfast during the 1970s embed themselves deeply and remain with me. I was visiting a vulnerable family in one such area and, on leaving their home, I assured them that I would return within a couple of days to reassess their situation and give them my continued support.

As promised, I did so, but on arrival in the neighbourhood I was unable to access the street because of an official security barrier at the entrance. Parking the car further along I retraced my steps and scrambled over the obstruction. To my amazement and horror, a large section of the entire row of terrace houses on both sides had been reduced to smouldering ruins – a casualty of the sectarianism rampant in that area at the time. I could not envisage which heap of rubble belonged to the family I was meant to be supporting.

In shock I must have stood transfixed at the spot for all of ten minutes until I think the security forces may have moved me on as an undesirable intruder. Despite efforts to trace them I never saw or heard of this family again. Disruption of continuity of care was a major problem for the healthcare team in the 1970s.**"**

Many dark days

A district nurse working in the same location relates her experience...

❝It was always my ambition to be a district nurse. I was delighted to be appointed to a post in Belfast in 1962. During the next few years, my working life was busy, rewarding and relatively normal. Unfortunately that normality would soon come to an abrupt end.

The advent of the period known as the Troubles wasn't a surprise to many as rumblings of discontent had been evident for some time. However the scale and duration of the Troubles could not have been imagined.

The darkest of many dark days for me began early on 9 August 1971. Having set off for work and not heard the news, I arrived on the Donegall Road/Falls Road in the midst of mayhem. Homes had been raided and men arrested. Many people were on the streets expressing and displaying their shock, anger and disbelief. Streets were blocked by barricades, vehicles were burning and rubble from rioting littered the streets alongside on-going sporadic violence. There was a strong army presence in the area.

I met up with a colleague and we decided to work and travel together that day in one car. We had great difficulty reaching our patients but we managed to do just that, despite many obstacles and a few punctures.

At this point I must say that at no time during this terrible day did we feel threatened or afraid. On the contrary, we were treated with kindness and respect by these poor people who in the midst of their fear and distress remained strong, offering help and support to their neighbours and ourselves. A cup of tea was always on offer and much appreciated. Their resilience made serving them an honour.

The following days, months and years held more of the same. One never knew what the next day held in store with something or somewhere provoking a spark for more violence.

Nursing in the community would continue to be problematic, however we continued to work and respond to all referrals on the same day. Co-operation between doctors, health visitors and social workers was excellent. The important role played by home helps must be recognised also, as their contribution to the care of the elderly and handicapped was invaluable.

I am all too often reminded these days by the news on television of unfortunate people in foreign parts fleeing their homes and countries carrying their belongings, so reminiscent of innocent people fleeing their homes in Bombay Street and New Barnsley. I remember clearly truck-loads of furniture and other belongings making their way along the streets of our city leaving behind burning homes and clouds of smoke.

It was like a scene from Gone with the Wind, but sadly this was no movie.

During the long troubled years we still had a job to do so we just got on with it; unbelievably we even got used to it.❞

Student nurses then and now

" *We were all oblivious to the challenges the next three years would bring."*

Student Nurse

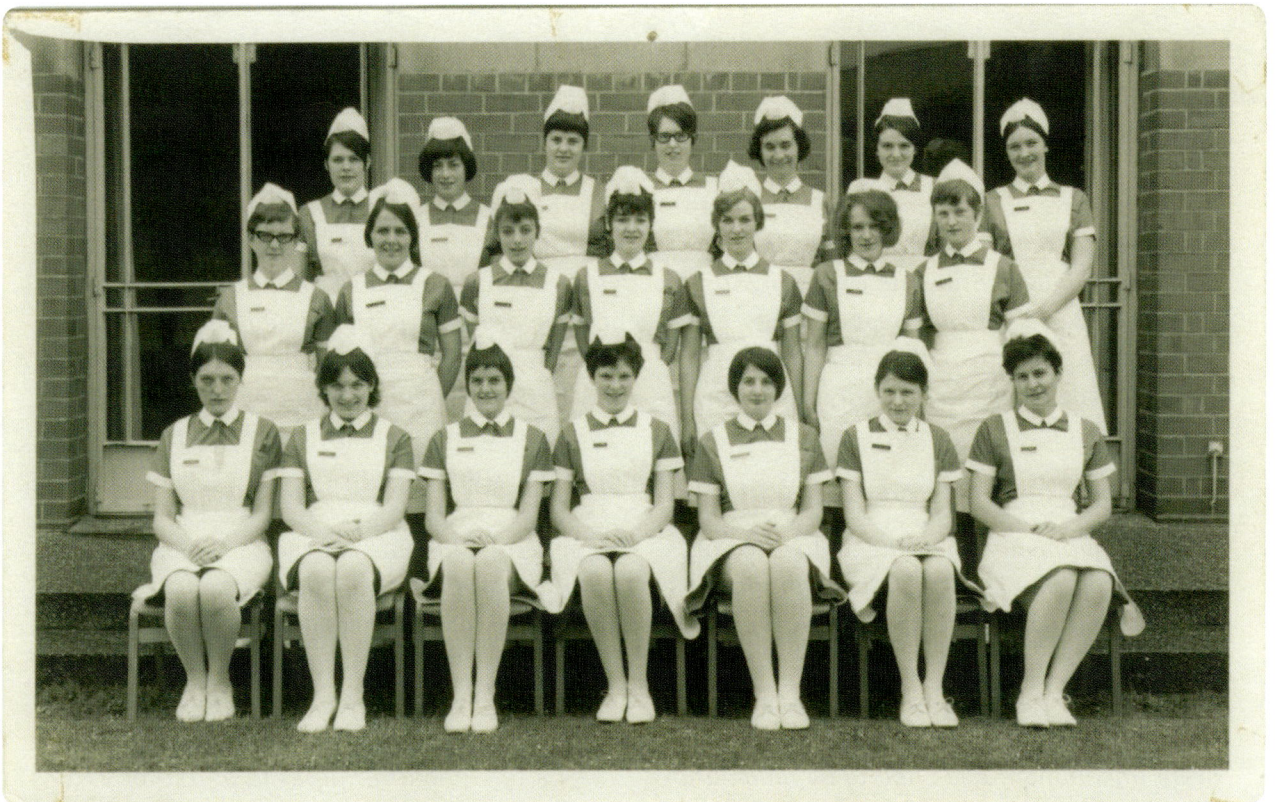

"Living on site bound us together…" Royal Victoria Hospital Preliminary Training School, 1969

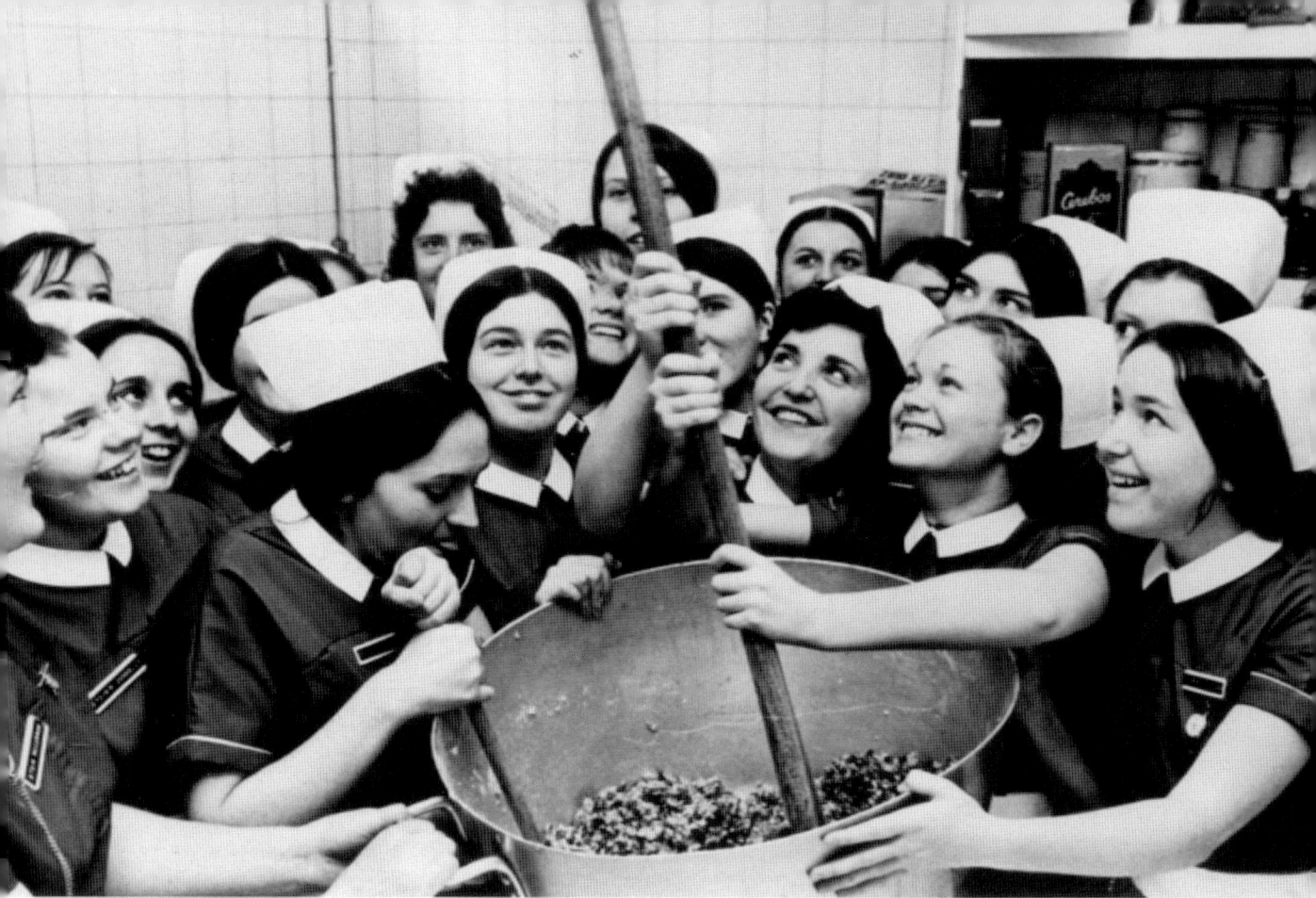

Stir-up Sunday, Belfast City Hospital, 1970s

When the Troubles started, nurse training was undertaken in most hospitals across Northern Ireland. Students were taught by senior nurses, with doctors giving lectures in their specialty. Unlike today, student nurses were paid staff and represented a large proportion of the workforce.

It was compulsory for students to "live-in" for most of their training. Accommodation usually was a small room just large enough to contain a single bed, wash-basin, chest of drawers and a wardrobe. Toilets and bath facilities were shared, shower facilities were uncommon. Beds had to be made and rooms left tidy for inspection by the home superintendent.

Many nurses' homes were locked for the night by 10pm. A nurse going off site and not due to return until after 10pm required a late pass. These were usually limited to three a month. Being single and remaining so for the duration of training was considered mandatory by most of the training schools.

In general, students obeyed the rules and regulations. There was no marked resistance to this boarding school regime even though this was the era of the swinging '60s, mini-skirts and flower power. However it was not unknown for nurses to climb drainpipes to a first- or second-floor bedroom window returning from a late night out!

While by modern-day standards this may all seem arcane and authoritarian, what came across strongly in gathering our stories were the bonds of friendship that developed in off-duty hours over tea and coffee in nurses' bedrooms.

For many nurses this is where they drew support to cope with the stresses of the day, which could range from encounters with the Ward Sister to dealing with horrific injuries. This was in fact the "counselling service" of that era.

The nursing system at this time was task-orientated and the Ward Sister dictated the care of patients. All nursing procedures for each patient were listed and every nurse, junior or senior, had allocated tasks. It was the responsibility of the senior student in charge in the absence of the Ward Sister to make sure all duties had been completed, even if it meant working past the designated "off-duty" time.

It was common practice for senior students to be left in charge of a general medical or surgical ward for an evening shift, and students were in charge at night under supervision of the night sister.

In the direst circumstances there was usually someone who had a funny story to tell to help ease anxiety and tensions. These informal gatherings were remembered with much affection and were seen to give the psychological support needed to get on with the next day's work. This is evident in the following stories from students and newly qualified nurses.

Supporting each other

❝I was in the May 1969 Preliminary Training School at the Royal Victoria Hospital (RVH) and we were thrown in at the deep end, so to speak, when the Troubles started later that year. We found ourselves experiencing some very turbulent and difficult times, and had to witness some horrifying and traumatic situations. But it was part of the package and you just got stuck in and kept going.

I think the fact that we lived on-site in the nurses' home bound us together as a group and we supported each other through all the ups and downs. At the end of our shifts we congregated in someone's room with our mugs of tea or coffee and our digestive biscuits or,

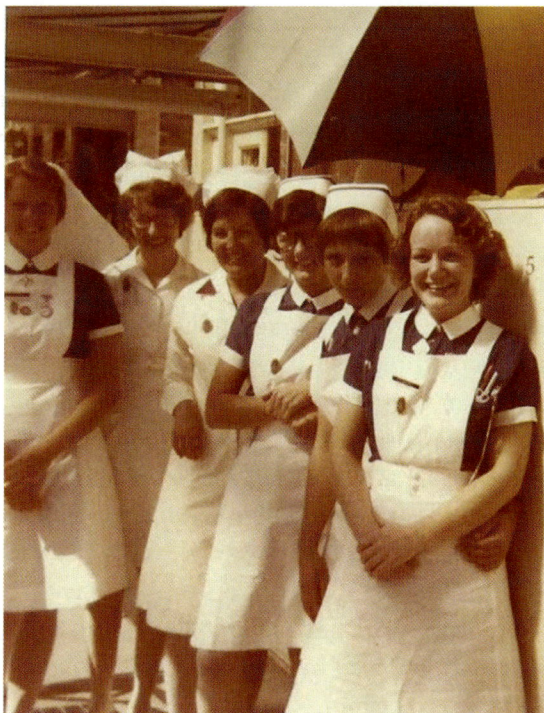

Nurses on RVH balcony, 1975

if we were lucky, some home-made flakemeal shortbread that had been sent from home. We talked about the things that had happened to us and got it out of our systems; we had some laughs too, and we survived!"

Introduction, induction, and initiation

"The year was 1972. I was 18 years old. My home was a farm by the sea in North Donegal, a beautiful, peaceful and rugged place. I left boarding school 'The Royal' in Raphoe in June and by September I had swapped one 'Royal' for another.

I had no real concept of the Troubles except perhaps a mention on the news on my parents' radio or television. I was more interested in my sport and my hockey, friends, fashion and the pop music of the day.

We were the September 1972 Preliminary Training School and in the main we were country girls or from smaller towns across the province.

Those early days in the nurse's home involved settling in, making new friends, and being prepared in the classroom by our tutors for our new lives as nurses. An initial challenge was learning how to put together that complicated student nurse's hat and to 'break in' our new white shoes.

For the first six weeks of our training we would live, work and sleep in Musson House, closely supervised by our wardens Mrs Black and Miss Copeland. The evenings were often spent relaxing in a small common room in the

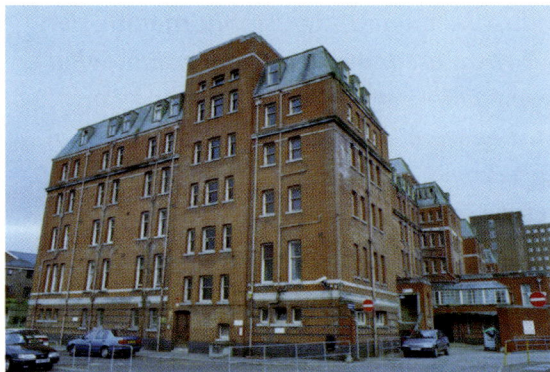
Musson House: "We laughed our way through drama."

basement of the home aptly named 'The Den'. It was a familiar routine in many ways as we were all essentially still schoolgirls.

We grew up quickly as, barely a week into our new lives, we were awakened one night by gunfire outside the nurses' home. I remember seeing lights flashing outside my bedroom window and the noise getting louder and louder. I stumbled out of bed and into the corridor to find my sleepy eyed, pyjama-clad colleagues asking each other what was happening.

Puzzled and perturbed we were told to lie on the corridor floor by the Belfast girls. They had experience of life in Belfast in the early 1970s and were considerably frustrated by our naivety.

Next day it was business as usual and 'don't tell your parents – we don't need to worry them'.

Thereafter we were to spend many more nights on the corridor floors until the worst of the shooting had passed. The advice from our wardens was 'remember girls, always keep two walls between you and the gunfire'.

We laughed our way through much of the drama. One of our group went to bed at night with rollers in her hair; they were kept in place by a pair of knickers, the hairnet of the day, and on one such occasion on the floor she was heard to say: 'If I get shot please take my knickers off my head before the ambulance comes!'

We became accustomed to gunmen in the hospital grounds, on the roof of the nurses' homes, and in and around the main hospital building. The army and police were never far away and as such at the time the hospital was seen as a legitimate target. Many such events went largely unreported as there were bigger and more catastrophic shootings and bombings occurring on a daily basis.

Shopping in Belfast was an important outing, deciding how to spend our monthly salary of £65. We had three choices in terms of travelling to the city centre: the Falls, or Grosvenor and Donegall roads – all regarded as equally dangerous. On one such outing a group of us were challenged while waiting at the Donegall Road bus-stop by young men from the area and asked if we were 'Taigs'? (Catholics). One of our group answered indignantly: 'No we are student nurses!' We were left alone after that unexpected response, but we debated this new addition to our vocabulary all the way to the city centre.

At the end of our six weeks' induction and classroom life, we celebrated with an event aptly known as the 'At Home'. Our parents were invited to join us and celebrate our readiness for ward duty and our future nursing career.''

An apron doubled as a shield

For some, their student nurse experiences are as vivid as if they had happened only yesterday, as the following story shows…

''It was a strange experience going into that room in Musson House for the first time in August 1972, opening the door and seeing the old sash window directly opposite, which looked out over the grassy slope towards the Children's Hospital.

Walking in to find the bed behind the door, wash-basin and small mirror on the opposite wall, I wondered what I was doing here. This bedroom was going to be my home for at least the next year and though I felt quite lonely and apprehensive, I consoled myself with the thought that I didn't really intend to stay that long. Just get enough money to go to Europe, that's what my friend Valerie and I had planned. She was already there and I was merely trying to earn some cash for the fare and initial living expenses. And that's how I arrived at Musson House to start my nursing career.

The building was not only the School of Nursing in those days, it was also the nurses' home at the Royal Victoria Hospital, Belfast. Walking into the room that day, I couldn't even begin to know how my life would change.

The day the uniforms arrived was a landmark event. There it was; the dress, the hat, the belt, the buckle, but the item which was to become the most significant was quietly lying to one side, wrapped in plastic. I opened it and began to unfold the material, and there it was, the white starched apron. I tried it on and it was stiff as a board. Little did I know then that this would become for me the symbol of a shield, something which would keep my pain in and allow me to function as if I was at all times in control.

Of course all of those who started nursing at that time had lived through the Troubles. The shootings, the bombings, the fear of going out just in case something happened. The July before I started I had been caught up in what is now known as 'Bloody Friday', when 22 bombs exploded all over Belfast. I had gone into Belfast to get some items I needed to start nursing and found myself in the middle of mayhem. I was one of the lucky ones to have returned home that day.

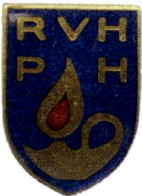

Staying strong

Back then I was a fun-loving, somewhat naïve 18 year old, but soon I was to face situations which tested me to the limit of my resilience. I learnt quickly not to speak of my own fear or pain at what I witnessed. Staying strong was the name of the game, using the white starched apron as a shield to absorb not only the blood and tears, but to keep my feelings firmly locked in, only to leak through as single tears in moments of complete emotional saturation.

I remember one of those occasions when I came close to the edge. It had been a terrible day and now as night rolled on, no one asked about going off-duty; it was too busy and ambulances had been arriving most of the evening. Apart from earlier trouble in the town, a prolonged gun battle was taking place and some of the wounded were rushed in. Casualty had two main areas, majors and minors, and both were crowded.

Police and army personnel were everywhere, members of the public were arguing and screaming at anyone in a uniform, hospital staff were running around. I was one of the juniors and I was trying desperately to be of help, but inwardly felt quite paralysed by what was going on in front of me. Suddenly my name was called and the nurse in charge told me to go to a cubicle and stay with a patient who was dying. She said no more could be done for him.

The man had been shot and a considerable portion of his skull was missing, his face was unrecognisable and there was blood and brain tissue everywhere. Covered in sheets and hooked up to an IV he lay there moaning and crying out. I went over to the trolley and told the patient my name and held his hand. He suddenly grasped it so hard I thought my hand would break and he slowly turned towards me.

I had never seen such wounds. He spoke incoherently and became frustrated when I couldn't understand. I eventually put my face down close to what was left of his and he asked me to pray. My uniform and apron were covered in blood and tissue and there, in the midst of mayhem, he grasped my hands and begged me to say a prayer. There we stayed, he and I, and spoke together to a higher being; each of us in our own way asking for divine intervention.

Gruesome tasks

Another night, I had just come on night duty. Handover given, I was assigned to 'special' a patient in the side ward who had sustained third-degree burns in a bombing incident. I made a note of what needed to be done during the night and went to the side ward to take over from the nurse already there. I opened the door and was shocked at what I saw in front of me.

The person in the bed was totally blackened, no hair of any kind, rather skeletal and almost unrecognisable as a human being. The thing I remember most was the smell of burnt flesh and, in the light of the dim Anglepoise light, the long night began. I had experience of dealing with people injured as a result of bombing and had been involved in the gruesome tasks of managing the large plastic bags which contained body parts gathered from bomb scenes. It was not until now that I had ever witnessed a human being so incinerated that the fact that life remained was in itself a mystery.

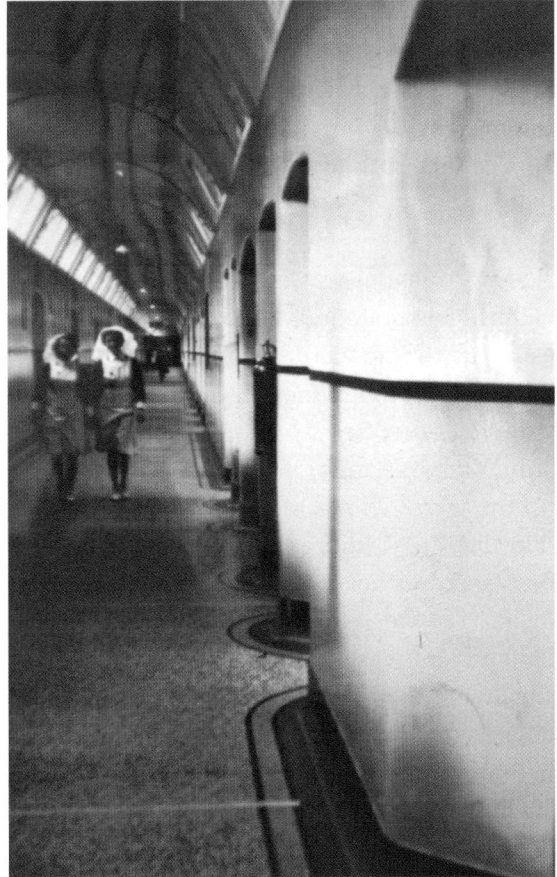

Royal Victoria Hospital main corridor, late 1960s

I spent the entire night with this poor man, trying to help ease his pain and just be with him. With one so critically injured not much else can be achieved. As dawn broke my patient, eventually after much trauma, silently left this world.

Keeping the peace

The corridor in the RVH was a highly significant place for those of us who worked there. The majority of wards led off from the main corridor and one always knew when duties started or ended by the swarm of nurses coming and going from each of the sets of black plastic doors which led to wards 1 to 20. Swinging through a set of doors one morning I walked the short distance to the next set leading into the ward proper, past the doctor's office, the clinical room, the side wards and into the Sister's office. There she was, the one in red, the one who must be obeyed… and generally feared! No happy affirming good morning, just a gruff incoherent grunt emanated from the powerful one. The morning report suggested a degree of concern in respect of four patients in particular. Nothing much to do with their physical wellbeing; more to do with the challenges of nursing in Northern Ireland.

Two of the four had been admitted the evening before, both with paramilitary backgrounds, one the result of trauma inflicted by the other. This had only become apparent to both of them at around 6am that morning.

The ward layout was based on the old Nightingale system of beds in rows along each side of the ward. One of the patients concerned lay three up on the left-hand side, the other two up on the right-hand side. The other pair of patients were further up the ward, which in those days suggested that they were improving sufficiently to now be placed further from the nursing station.

One patient was a devout Roman Catholic (RC) with a liberal display of religious objects surrounding him. The other, who patently did not subscribe to the Roman Catholic faith, had begun an argument with the first patient, and a loud and rather aggressive row ensued. Sister put me in charge of the 'male side' and as I looked up the ward I wondered how well the 'shield' (my apron) would do today. I have of course since learned that nothing is so bad that it can't get worse and when relatives of all four patients arrived stamina was required.

Sister swung into action and delegated me to deal with the patients whilst she endeavoured to manage the relatives. Without doubt the red dress had its effect and relatives were duly calmed, I began moving my patients around the area to facilitate a more peaceful environment. Though I did receive complaints that by using side areas I was 'giving in' to unreasonable demands that attitude

changed later. The peace was also assisted by one of the patient's relatives bringing in numerous flower bouquets, which were placed on the table at the end of the bed so that he did not have to look at the patient opposite.

A busy evening shift
I was on a 2pm-5pm split shift that particular day and, returning to the ward at 5pm, I thought that the worst that could happen that evening was that the relatives would all reappear at visiting time and a microcosm of the Northern Ireland Troubles would recommence.

That wasn't to be as, later that evening, a major incident took place in which nine people were admitted straight from casualty to the ward with gunshot wounds. Each patient required to be prepared for theatre and amidst the business of ensuring readiness for theatre, beds needed to be moved again and those who had previously argued became subdued.

Managing people in fear of losing their life and in extreme pain, traumatised by what has happened to them, has a lasting effect on all who come in contact. Though busy, each patient needed time to speak, to be reassured, to cry, to be with another human being and tell the story of what had happened. My 'shield' absorbed so much pain that evening that when eventually I came off duty at 1am I walked very, very slowly up the long black corridor to Bostock canteen and tried very hard not to cry, hoping that tonight there would be no gun battles around the nurses' home.

The bomber

Another day I was assigned to a really busy orthopaedic, 84-bed unit. The top end of the unit was the secure area where specific patients were guarded by police, who in turn were guarded by the army. Next section were bays dedicated to those patients who had sustained pelvic or upper leg fractures; the next set of bays had patients who were mostly those injured in shootings or bombings and the last set of bays were normally for those with sporting injuries.

All patients with different physical and psychological needs, all displaying fortitude during the day, but sometimes at night their true pain revealed itself.

I was on night duty and on coming out of the lift and walking towards the nursing station, I met some day staff whose facial expressions and words of warning made me consider getting back into the lift and going away. However, I went on and instinctively put my hands inside the top of my apron, just ensuring that the real me stayed firmly inside the starch.

Report was relatively normal except for a new patient admitted that evening from theatre who was in a critical state. He wasn't from Northern Ireland and his family were en route by boat and scheduled to arrive later. He had been involved in an explosion, no one else injured; he had apparently been preparing a bomb when it had gone off prematurely. After report I went to check on him. His injuries were extensive. He had lost legs, one arm, one eye, and had extensive facial and torso injuries. He was 21 years old, had a one-year-old daughter and came from a family of two sisters and one other brother. He had come to help the 'cause' and had told his family he was coming to stay in Northern Ireland for a few days with friends.

I sat with him as he drifted in and out of post-anaesthetic sleep; he was practically mute with trauma and in extreme pain and, given his injuries and general lack of reasonable tissue, maintaining patency in IV infusions was going to be difficult. I have never forgotten this patient, who was just a year older than I.

Though I had witnessed suffering more or less continually throughout those awful years of the 1970s, the sound of what could only be described as a primordial cry that emanated from his mother when she first saw him has never left me.

Another long slow walk up the black corridor to Bostock coming off duty next morning, watching porters and trolleys, goods vans arriving, the acute sting of sunlight in your eyes – only felt by those coming off night duty – everything apparently normal. But it wasn't. Nothing was normal. 🥢

A second-year student remembers…

Shiny black boots

❝An army Land Rover had been involved in an incident near to the hospital. Staff in casualty had been alerted to the arrival of injured personnel. I remember being in resuscitation and feeling nervous as the trolleys of injured were wheeled in.

I was kept busy getting different items needed. I remember being asked to get a drug out of the cupboard and as I turned to bring it to the person in charge I noticed a trolley covered with a sheet. It was apparently a young soldier who was 18 years old, nearly the same age as me. I remember his black shiny boots protruding out from under the white sheet that covered his body. I thought about the time he took to get such a sheen and how proud he must have been going on duty.

My late night call-up
During the time I worked in theatre, I was getting ready to go to bed one night when there was a knock at the door and I was asked to go back on duty. There had been a bomb blast and many people had been injured. On arriving in theatre I was shocked to see all the activity. It was different from any of the busy days that I had experienced there. I stood beside a man, trying to say the right things to help him feel less frightened. He talked about his legs being very painful. I felt frightened for him as he seemed to have horrific injuries.

I spent the night until about 4am doing all the jobs that a junior student can do. I watched surgeons and senior nursing staff work together with great skill. I was told to go back to bed at about 4am and return for duty in the morning as usual. I can't remember walking back to my room but I do remember coming on duty in the morning and one theatre had been made ready for use. I was asked to scrub for the removal of an appendix.

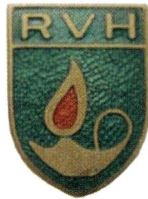

This poor man had been admitted as an emergency during the night but he had to wait. Sister told me she had been up all night and was still trying to get things sorted in theatres. She put me into the capable hands of the surgeon and told him this was my first time to assist on my own. Mr Willoughby Wilson led me, as a first-timer, through the operation in a kind and gentle manner.❞

I grew older overnight

A first-year student nurse recollects…

❝He was the first black man that I ever touched. Later I would work as a nurse in Africa (1987-2010), but I have often thought back to the night when the soldier arrived in recovery ward in the Royal Victoria Hospital.

He was caught up in a war that made distinctions between Protestant and Catholic, Unionist and Nationalist, but not between black and white. What did this handsome man have to do with our home-grown conflict?

I was on night duty in the recovery ward on 31 May 1972. We were not long into our shift when an enormous explosion rocked the building and rattled the windows. The evenings were light until late and we were able to look out of the recovery ward windows up above the main corridor. We could see clouds of ominous smoke rising from Springfield Road Police Station where there was also an army base.

Almost immediately ambulances with sirens blaring rushed out of the hospital gates towards the scene of the explosion. We knew that it was going to be another demanding night in the theatres of the Royal and in our recovery ward. It was a night that this 19-year-old student nurse would remember clearly for years to come.

He arrived into casualty and was rushed to theatre. From there he was brought to the recovery ward. 'He is unconscious. The surgeon did not operate,' we were told by the reporting nurse. 'He has bad internal injuries including head injuries. Just make him as comfortable as possible.'

With this terse report, the nurse in charge asked me to stay with him till he died. A portable screen was put around his bed. I felt helpless. I wanted to do something to help him, but what could I do? Even his name spoke of a different culture and origin than my own. I wondered about his family far away. Did they know he was dying? I remember looking down at his shoulder muscles and strong body still covered with a white coating of dust from the explosion.

I filled a basin of warm water and, as best I could without disturbing him, I washed the dust from his face, lashes and thick curly hair. I cleaned his broad shoulders. I held his strong hand and talked to him as I gently adjusted his pillow. I wanted him to know he was not alone. Within an hour he slipped away from this life still unaware of the 30lb bomb that had wrecked the police station and cut short his life at 28 years of age.

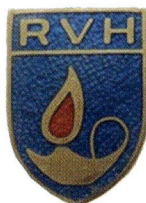

Later I learned that he was a very popular army lightweight boxing champion who had represented Ulster and England. His roots were in the Seychelles. He had a wife and four children. I am glad that he was not alone when he died in our war.

Coming off night duty was tough that next morning. In contrast to day duty, there were no other nurses available to listen to my personal traumas of the night. I felt like I had grown older overnight. I had been through something most young women do not have to cope with in a life-time. But telling my part in this soldier's story would have to wait.

A year later

It was a regular summer day in August 1973 when I walked from Victoria Towers past the army base at Broadway to go on duty for a 1pm-9pm shift. I was a second-year student nurse on ward 16 in the Royal Victoria Hospital's main corridor. But the events of my 'ordinary' day have been etched into my memory ever since.

At the handover in the nurses' station I was told that my duty that day was to stay with a 29-year-old man. He had been handling explosive material when the incendiary device detonated prematurely. Staff Nurse explained that he had third degree burns over most of his body. Due to the fluid loss from the burns, shock and risk of infections, his condition was critical. His comrade, a young woman only 19 years old, was in the side ward off ward 15. She also had extensive burns.

It was with some trepidation that I entered the room, a small side-ward off ward 16. I had seen burns before when working in casualty, but this was in a different category. This man was charred black from head to toe. In the true 'get-on-with-it' approach ingrained into student nurses in the early 1970s, I thought: 'I can do this!'

But I was not prepared for the over-powering smell of burned flesh within the poorly ventilated confines of this tiny room. As the hours passed, the walls of the room seemed to increasingly crowd in on me. At times my head swooned and the nausea was about to engulf me. And yet I was determined not to give up.

I knew that my patient was dying. But I did my best to care for him: changing the IV fluids to replace what was oozing though his burns; keeping his eye pads moist to ease his discomfort and regularly giving him analgesic injections with the aim of keeping him as comfortable as possible. I gazed though the windows above his bed and prayed for God to have mercy on his soul. The minute hand on my lapel watch crawled on at a snail's pace. I tried not to count the hours until I would be released.

The door was kept closed and the noises of regular ward life were distant. A soldier with a machine gun was stationed outside the room – part of normal life in the main corridor of the Royal.

I remember feeling nothing but compassion for this young man. He was only ten years older than me and yet his life was over. A priest came and prayed. Concerned relatives came and went. I had no idea what to say to them. I stood beside his bed, holding his charred hand. I talked to him in a gentle voice knowing that his hearing might be still acute despite his injuries and sedation.

Late in the afternoon the consultant, Mr George Johnston, came to see his patient. After spending a few minutes in the room Mr Johnston turned to the nurse in charge and said, 'Do not keep this young nurse in here for her entire shift. Arrange for someone to relieve her now and then.' Mr Johnston had seen my pallid face and read the situation with concern for me. He was like an angel to me that day. The short breaks I was given during my eight-hour shift helped me through that long, emotionally demanding day. Even today when I smell burned meat, memories of this day flood back.

Coming off-duty to the nurses' home was almost always therapeutic. A group of girls would gather in one room or flat with coffee, tea, toast and biscuits, and relate their tales of the day. We had no formal debriefing. No one talked of post-traumatic stress disorder during those years. We informally debriefed each other and got on with the job that we were trained to do. We were all in this heart-wrenching conflict together and even though we were very young we felt proud of our professionalism and steadfastness.

My patient died a week later. His female colleague died two days later. They were nursed with the same diligent care we gave all our patients, without any discrimination according to religion or political views."

My first scrub

A student nurse in theatres remembers…

"I looked forward to my theatre placement as the area behind the 'red line' where patients were transferred for surgery into the care of the theatre team had an aura of mystery and importance. My placement there was during the summer months of my second year of training.

I began my theatre experience at the start of the 12th of July holiday fortnight and was disappointed to learn that planned surgery was not scheduled for part of the holiday period; instead the main job to be completed was routine spring cleaning. How mundane!

We scrubbed, counted and inspected instruments in the different surgical packs which were sterilised by the central sterile supplies department. We were taught the names and use of different instruments. We were also shown how to scrub up for assisting as the scrub nurse to hand instruments and swabs to the surgeon.

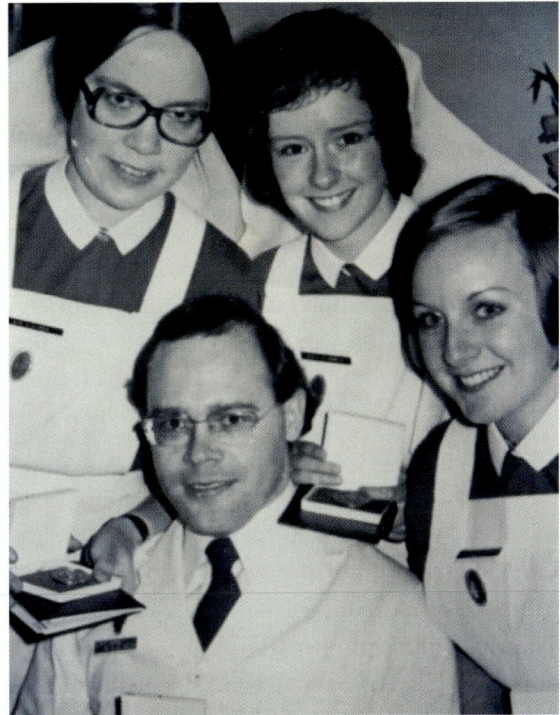

Newly qualified nurses, 1974

I don't remember the lead up to the afternoon I found myself scrubbed to assist with the possible amputation of a leg following an injury to a member of the security forces. I knew nothing of the circumstances which had resulted in the casualty.

My first memory is standing beside an instrument trolley at the foot of a theatre table on which lay the casualty. In my mind's eye I still see teams of surgeons and gowned nurses. It was clear that the injuries sustained were to head and abdomen as well as legs. I remember methodically counting out swabs. More senior nurses were there as assistant 'runners' to fetch any additional requirements. The person lying on the theatre table seemed huge and I assumed that if he had come that far there was hope of survival after the surgery to be carried out. My heart was in my stomach, as I didn't want to be making any blunders. This was my first scrub. There were no familiar or reassuring faces around, and even if there were, everyone was masked and gowned. I recognised nobody. I just remember keeping myself busy counting swabs, when I sensed an arm motioning me to stop.

I looked around the table and all the teams had stopped and stepped back from the theatre trolley. Everyone was standing in silence, nobody moved, heads were bowed. Then I heard a continuous sobbing coming from the outside corridor. This was the security guard grieving at the loss of a colleague. It was only then that I fully realised the patient had died on the table.

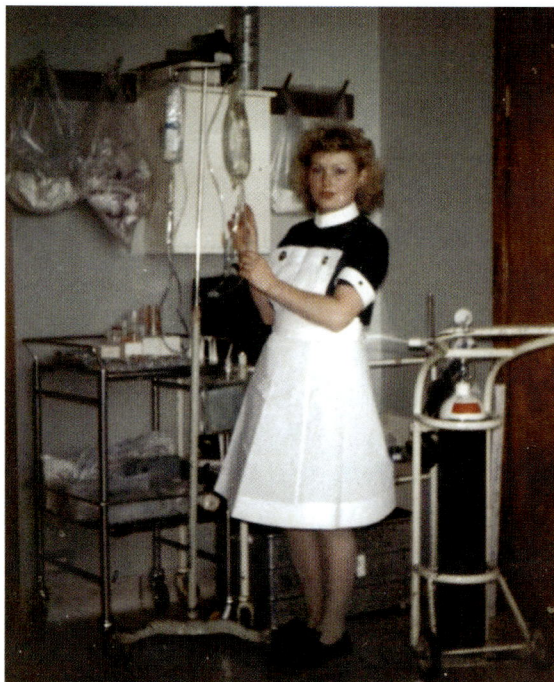

Altnagelvin nurse with portable drip, 1970s

I did not find out until much later that there had been other deaths associated with this particular incident. I still do not know who the casualty was but I will never forget the echo of those sobs from his colleague which drifted around theatre.

That experience of a patient the same age as me dying on the theatre table was horrific. I have no recollection of descrubbing or the remainder of that shift. There was no counselling then and I lived out, sharing a rented house with best friends. I can't

remember if I discussed this with them, I certainly never told my parents as I didn't want them to be alarmed or worried about what I was being exposed to. Also we were always reminded about the confidentiality of our patients. Thankfully afterwards I had the opportunity of scrubbing for planned, everyday procedures such as gall bladder removal and so on and theatre for me resumed its normality. However the memory of my first scrub will stay with me forever. **"**

So many duties

"Having left school a few months earlier, I soon discovered that the duties of a very junior nurse were seemingly endless.

Around Christmas 1971, in a surgical ward in the Royal, I stood behind the screens at the bedside of an elderly man and tears ran down my face. We had just received the morning report and allocation of duties. I was overwhelmed with the realisation that every task seemed to have been allocated to me!

Some patients needed to be taken for a walk; others required oral fluids hourly with careful documentation of quantities. Several required mouth-care every four hours and regular turning. There were patients to be admitted and all their valuables, to the last coin, had to be recorded and carefully made safe. Ten o'clock teas had to be prepared and given out. Trays had to be prepared for lunch. The list went on and on.

As my tears continued to flow, the elderly patient, the owner of a Belfast chip shop, looked on with concern. Thankfully, a very caring and efficient State Enrolled Nurse came to my rescue. She assured me that the responsibility did not all lie on my shoulders.

I recall there was a mix of patients in that long and busy Nightingale ward. There were those recovering from elective surgery as well as patients with injuries associated with Troubles. Members of the security forces and paramilitaries lay side-by-side, often gravely ill.

One senior member of the security forces, possibly in his forties, was recovering from gunshot wounds to his abdomen. One day, as he walked from the toilet to his bed, pushing his drip-stand, he began to shake violently. As I helped him into bed, I had no idea what was happening. I soon learned that this was a rigor and was the result of a severe reaction to his intravenous infusion. He recovered well.

Sometime after his discharge, I bumped into him again in a café in County Tyrone. He recounted to my mother and aunt the good nursing care that he had received while injured: 'Nobody knows the good work that those wee girls do.' When my family was ready to leave the café, we found that our bill had been paid. If this patient happens to read this story, thank you very much!

A bullet in the linen cupboard
On one of my first weeks of night duty as a student nurse I was on the metabolic ward, a block adjacent to the main corridor of the Royal.

There was a commotion one evening, just as I was arriving, due to a bullet being fired into the linen cupboard on the first floor. The shot was apparently fired from the top of the School of Dentistry. The handover report was obviously delayed, as senior hospital staff arrived, along with senior army personnel.

I made my way to the second floor to where I had been assigned for the week. There was an anxious silence about the ward, but no sense of panic. Miss Gaw, the Night Superintendent, was concerned about my welfare and moved my desk, chair and mandatory Anglepoise lamp away from the window. Clearly health and safety at work must be maintained! However the risk assessment did not take account of the fact that we were still in the firing line and evacuation, as far as I know, was never contemplated.

We had become familiar with gunfire in the early weeks of our training at the Royal; the sound of bullets whizzing past the nurses' home was not uncommon. However, the inherent danger never occurred to us. We just kept a low profile, in fact as low as possible – I remember one frightening occasion spent sheltering on the floor. **"**

Keep calm and carry on

"I was doing midwifery in the Jubilee Maternity Hospital around 1971-1972.

We had to go to the YMCA Hall in Belfast city centre to sit our first part written examination. During that morning there were three explosions in the city. I recall after each one how the invigilators spoke to us, telling us to remain calm and carry on. They kept very calm themselves. It must have been difficult as, after the third explosion, many candidates became very anxious.

It was a frightening experience and I was very glad to escape from that hall and, with others, quickly make my way back to the sanctuary of the hospital.

Needless to say, our plans for having lunch out downtown were thwarted. **"**

Footsteps on the roof

A children's nurse remembers…

"One night I arrived on duty as a second-year student nurse. I was in charge of a 50-bed ward, with two first-year students and an auxiliary to care for all the children in the ward.

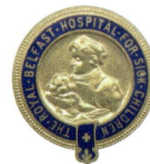

About an hour into the shift the night sister came round to say she had been told that the paramilitaries were taking over the Children's Hospital and we had to 'take precautions'. We heard running footsteps on the roof but didn't know whether they were soldiers or paramilitaries.

We had to black out the windows with thick blankets, pull all cots and beds away from the windows and move the babies from the nursery into the main ward.

It was an eerie night of listening to the footsteps running across the roof, hearing shots from time to time and trying to move around the ward with minimal lighting in order to carry out the care required for the children.

Because the shooting continued into the morning we weren't allowed back to the nurses' home so we had to take theatre gowns and we were given beds on the third floor of the Children's Hospital.

Another night we were in the nursery of the medical ward, which had a rather flimsy door leading into the car park at the front of the hospital and facing the Falls Road. We were in the milk kitchen making up feeds when this tremendous noise started out on the road. Through the window we could see crowds of people with bin lids banging on the road and shouting.

I found this very frightening as it continued for so long into the night. We moved the children from the nursery for safety and tried to reassure older children in the ward. It was a long and frightening night. **"**

Pink slippers

"In accident and emergency one Saturday night we were told a gunshot victim was coming. To this day I can still picture this scene.

This was a 60-year-old woman in a pink dressing gown and pink fur-lined slippers to match. I could picture her having had her Saturday night bath – one bath a week in those days – then into her bed attire. Well, there was a knock on her door and as she answered it, gunfire knocked her to the ground.

When she arrived with her wee husband, she was conscious and talking. Some blood could be seen on her chest area. As I cut off her clothes to investigate, she deteriorated and died. We sent her husband home alone giving him some diazepam.

The memory of that man's face is still etched in my mind's eye. Very traumatic. **"**

Heart surgery at short notice

A newly qualified staff nurse recalls how a patient recovered from his operation more quickly than she did...

"My first post after qualifying as an SRN was in operating theatres. One afternoon the ward staff advised us of a sudden deterioration in a newly admitted gunshot patient. This was an accidental discharge of a legally-held firearm, an event which was not uncommon, given the numbers of legally-held firearms in the province.

He had an abdominal entry wound, with no corresponding exit. I was the scrub nurse for the operation, responsible for handing the surgeon his instruments at the right time in the right order. Following anaesthetic, the surgeon opened the abdomen and rapidly inspected the interior. There was no bullet to be found, and no major injury.

Then came a laconic announcement from the anaesthetist at the top of the table: 'His blood pressure is dropping.' After that things began to happen rather quickly. The surgeon, a World War Two veteran who had cut his teeth with the wounded at Dunkirk, instinctively knew what the problem was. 'I'm going to do a thoracotomy,' he said.

Everyone seemed to know what was going to happen next – except this greenhorn Staff Nurse. Sister glided to my elbow and shot a suture onto my sterile Mayo tray. 'I'm giving you a 2/0 silk on a round-bodied needle,' she murmured. 'Use a long-handled needle holder.' Out of the corner of my eye I saw sterile defibrillator paddles being passed over the anaesthetic screen for use directly on the heart if required. A number of blood units were now being transfused simultaneously, the anaesthetist squeezing the bags to speed up the rate.

The next thing I saw was the mediastinum open, and heart muscle flailing wildly within the cavity. With every rapid beat, a jet of blood leapt out of the wound. The abdominal entrance wound had been misleading. The bullet had in fact traversed the chest, and the patient was rapidly losing blood through a hole in the heart wall.

Without a word the surgeon took the suture. With a few deft movements he sewed the bullet wound closed. Blood loss was now arrested, and the crisis was over. He then located and retrieved the bullet, checking it had done no further damage.

This highly dangerous situation left me shell-shocked, and I cannot recall the rest of the operation. Afterwards, when the surgeon had completed his notes, I took the file round to the post-op ward. There the patient was already sitting up talking to his relatives. He was making a more rapid recovery than this scrub nurse.

This episode significantly reinforced the existing respect I had for my seniors in surgery and nursing. I had just seen proof that the hospital was a precise and well-oiled machine that could rise effortlessly to any challenge which presented itself. It could even master life-saving heart surgery at short notice. And I was now a small part of it.**"**

A hierarchical system

A Mater Hospital student nurse recalls how Matron, a nun, ran the hospital like a battleship…

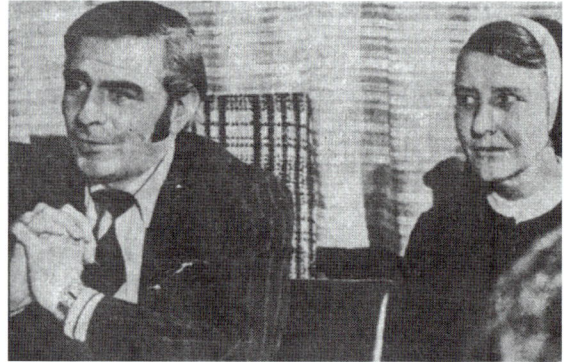

Pat Kinder and Sister Ignatius, Mater Hospital

"Working in the Mater Hospital in Belfast during the early Troubles was a unique environment. The unit had been run by the Sisters of Mercy as an independent hospital since its inception in the late 19th century and had only become part of the NHS in the early 1970s.

For many years it continued to retain a strong religious culture with a hierarchical management system, was highly regimented and in many ways felt like a girls' boarding school. We all lived together, we worked together and we played together.

The emotional security provided by this environment probably played a very important role in how many of us as 17- and 18-year-old girls coped with the traumatic events we were facing daily. We had a wonderful, tough, authoritative matron, a nun called Sister Ignatius, who ran the hospital like a battleship. She knew every patient and member of staff and ensured everyone delivered standards of care which would be the envy of any healthcare trust today. There were many challenges – multiple bomb blast victims, gunshot wounds, exposure to personal threats and violence on a routine basis, and fear for our personal safety. We always felt we were targets; Catholic nurses in a Catholic hospital in a loyalist area.**"**

Standards must be maintained

"There was a breed of woman in the Royal Victoria Hospital that was quite unlike any other. They were truly women of substance. Many occupied senior nursing management positions, many held 'red' sister posts, while many others were domestics and cleaners.

In the 1970s, none of the assistant matrons or night superintendents were married, not necessarily by choice. Marriage and career were mutually exclusive states for senior nurses in those days. Amongst the mayhem these women brought order, or denial, whichever way one chooses to interpret it.

One night I was on duty on the 'corridor' and it was unbelievably busy. Thankfully no major incidents were coming through the door, just the normal busy of any large hospital. I was the staff nurse in charge. I had washed my hair before coming on duty and tied it up so it would fit neatly inside my 'fall'. This was the diamond-shaped veil we wore to tell the world we were now

qualified nurses. No matter how many clips I put into my hair that evening, my fall continually slipped and found its way down my back. The stud I had in my starched collar was also giving me grief; I'd lost the straight stud and was forced to resort to the butterfly variety which I hated. Everything pointed to it being a bad night.

It began: central venous pressure lines started playing up, the condition of four patients deteriorated within a relatively short space of time. IV drips went into the tissues and had to be dealt with. The fall slid further and further down my back.

Calmness restored for a short while, then a patient went into cardiac arrest. Unlike today the beds in those days didn't move up and down. Those of us somewhat vertically challenged had to find ingenious ways of administering cardiopulmonary resuscitation. So while colleagues contacted the arrest team I climbed up on the bed and began to attempt to resuscitate the patient. 'Ping!' – that was the sound of the butterfly stud breaking, the fall gave up and floated to the ground – just in time the resus team arrived and thankfully the patient was successfully resuscitated.

'Well done,' said the doctor in charge, 'you did a great job there.'

Walking down the ward, fall in hand, open collar, stud broken, my eyes were drawn to the lady in blue walking up the ward. Hat perfect, lace collar, eyes glaring in my direction.

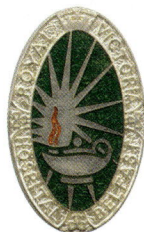

'Are you in charge?' with an emphasis on the word 'you', which suggested either disbelief or incredulity.

Trying to grapple with the collar and randomly clip the fall back in place I replied I was. Then it came: not 'well done' or 'busy night, have you had a break, everything okay?' No, not for these women. They demanded total professionalism, no wimps allowed! I was informed I had two minutes to rearrange my uniform, collar studded, fall in place, apron straps crossed at mid-point on the back. During that two minutes Matron would check the ward to ensure that all was well.

Was this hard and insensitive? No, it was keeping us focused on the job in hand, reminding us that no matter what happened, we maintained standards.

I was back in two minutes; sorted, with the help of a paper clip for the collar and 20 grips in my hair I was inspected. Apparently having passed, just one more query: 'Are you Royal-trained?'"

Canny management

"When I began training in 1971, Matron and her deputies were viewed by nurses with a mixture of respect and fear. They all had long practical experience as ward sisters and as administrators, and were battle-hardened after the first few years of the Troubles.

They took it in turn to do standby overnight in west wing in the hospital, overlooking the Grosvenor Road and within sight and sound of the conflict just outside the walls.

One of their roles was to ensure adequate staffing at short notice especially after major incidents. In 1972 our nursing class was in school during a period of particularly heavy demand. Day after day the Deputy Matron, Miss May McFarland, arrived seeking volunteers to go on ward duty after class.

'Mac' was a canny Fermanagh woman, and it was only after her generation had retired that I came to appreciate her shrewd hands-on management style. Mac didn't circulate memos – she got out of her office, visited the scene, talked in her brisk homely tones to the right people, and obtained rapid results.

After a few weeks of regular demand our class eventually wearied of volunteering. One nurse protested: 'But we are entitled to our time off!' That weekend one of our own hospital professionals, Janet Bereen, had been killed in the city-centre Abercorn bomb attack. 'Janet was entitled to her time off too!' came the tart response. Mac got her volunteers, and there was no more quibbling.

One night in the 1970s at a hospital lecture in Bostock Ballroom, I noticed the theatre nursing officer walking the aisle and scanning the audience. She was on the lookout for theatre nurses, myself being one of them. Just after teatime two factions of the IRA had gone to war with one another, and casualty was now chock-a-block with gunshot wounds. I accepted her invitation to depart with some readiness.

Producing extra hands at short notice required fine managerial judgement. Suddenly allocating more nurses to work overnight inevitably depleted numbers next day, with the potential to disrupt routine surgery. The skill was to match the emergency workload with sufficient numbers – and no more.

One Sunday morning in the 1980s in fracture clinic I realised the hospital was running out of beds. There was never enough room in the fracture wards for our manifold casualties, and I constantly needed to borrow spaces from ward sisters throughout a very large hospital complex. It was unprecedented that we should have no empty beds, so I duly notified my medical and nursing superiors of an impending crisis.

That afternoon I failed to find a bed for a trauma admission, so once again I rang nursing administration and spoke to one of the experienced assistant matrons. 'My dear, this hospital has never run out of beds,' she said soothingly. 'Not even during the worst days of the Troubles.' She gave me a tip that the Eye Hospital was under-used at weekends. I contacted an ophthalmic surgeon via his ward sister, and he granted a bed. My problem was solved in ten minutes."

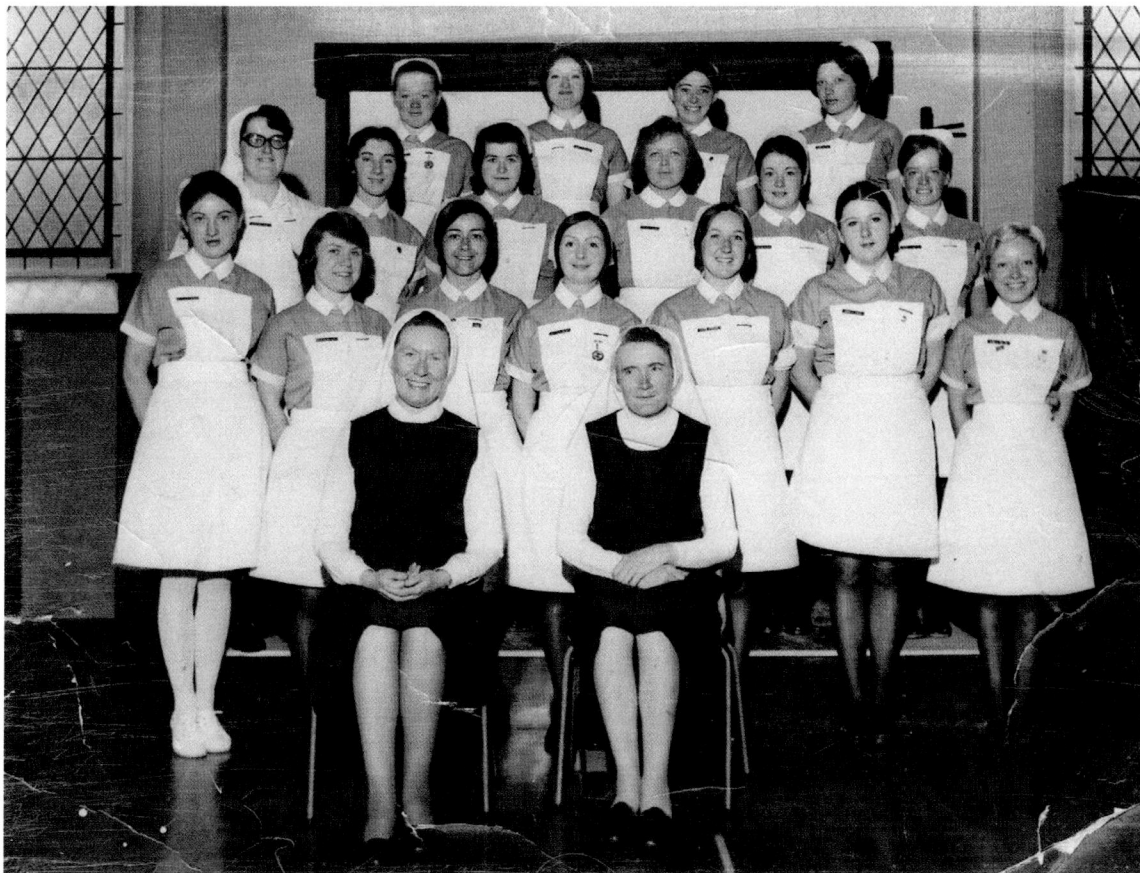

Mater Hospital, Preliminary Training School, 1971

Paramilitary punishments

"You wouldn't do this to a dog. This is the sort of thing you would see in medieval times, not today."

Patient's father

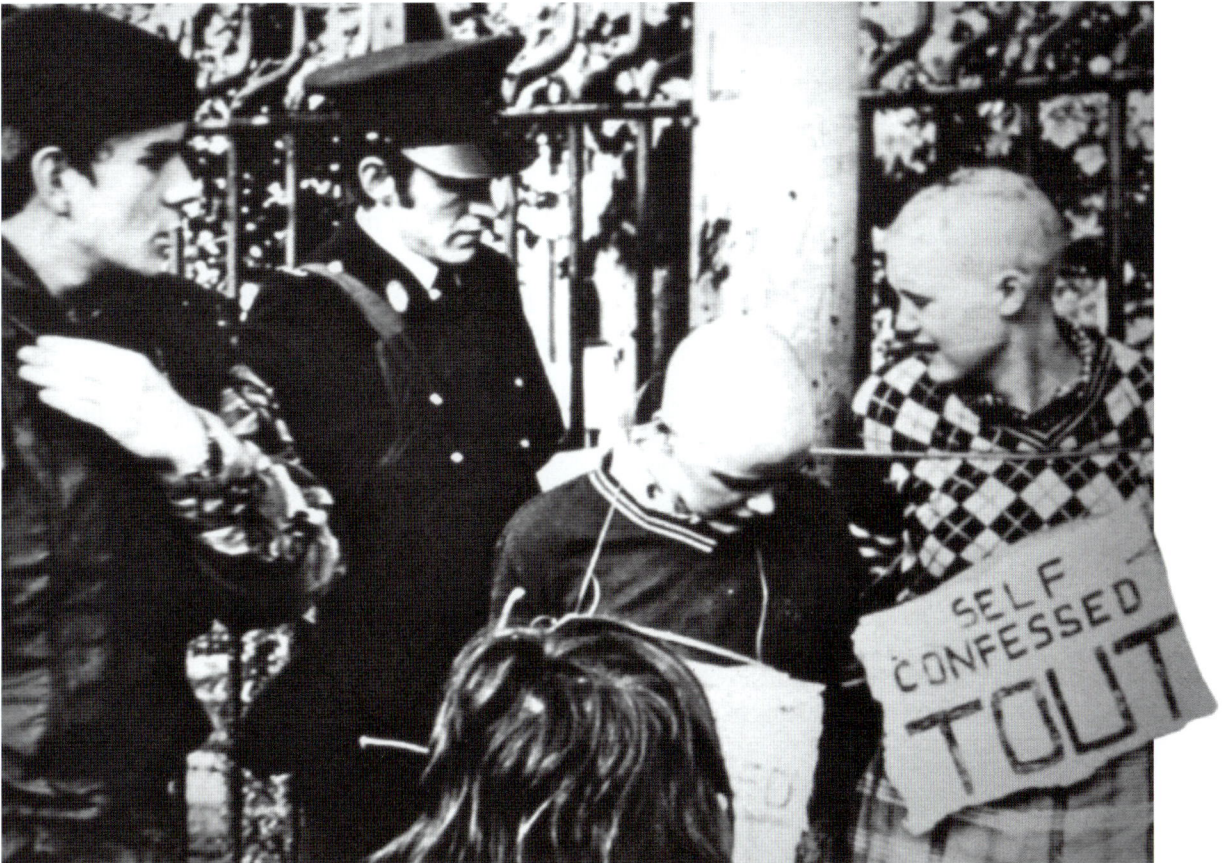

Victims were publicly humiliated

Caring for casualties of paramilitary punishment

By 2008 it was estimated that since the Troubles started there had been 6,404 punishment shootings and beatings.[1] Paramilitary punishments continued. These victims required time-consuming surgical treatment and care in hospital.

Nurses have described treating and caring for victims who were "tarred and feathered" or "kneecapped".

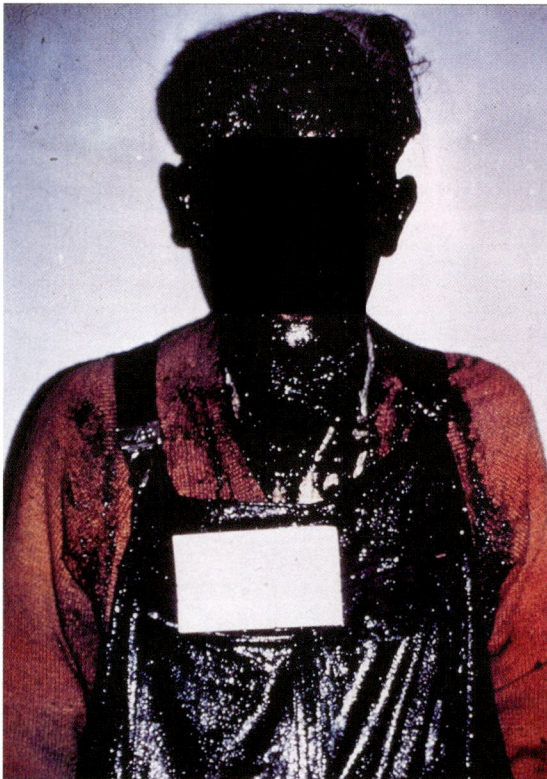

Man tarred, 1970: removal was a traumatic process

[1] Williams J (2005) Crime and punishment. Emergency Nurse. 13, 8.

[2] Steele-Nicholson A (1984) The Belfast Fixator. Nursing Times. 80, 8.

This was a form of punishment used by paramilitary organisations to humiliate victims considered to have acted outside of what was perceived as acceptable behaviour for the community in which they lived. Victims were publicly abused and had their head shaved before being covered in tar and feathers.

Some of these victims were so badly beaten and wounded beforehand that they required admission to theatre to remove the tar and treat the underlying injuries. Since the Ceasefire this form of punishment has largely died out.

Kneecapping was, and continues to be, a form of punishment carried out by paramilitary groups. Victims have allegedly committed antisocial behaviour such as joyriding or drug dealing.

Kneecapping methods vary depending on the perceived seriousness of the "crime". Victims may have bullets fired into their knees from front to back or side to side. The line of fire causes different severity of damage to arteries and bone. Some victims have additional wounds inflicted to their arms and ankles, sometimes referred to as a "six-pack". Other weapons known to have been used are drills, sticks and clubs.

During the early years of the Troubles, admissions of such victims to the Royal Victoria Hospital were so numerous that surgeons developed specialist techniques to treat the injuries.[2] In some cases the damage done was so severe that amputation was required.

Such patients underwent surgery from two hours upwards. One victim of such punishment required ten hours of surgery.

Most victims were young males who often repeated the "crime" they had been punished for and many were "punished" on more than one occasion.

The following stories are from nurses who cared for such patients...

Being "summoned"

❝I worked in the A&E department in Belfast City Hospital from 1982-2000, first as a staff nurse and then as charge nurse. During that time I was involved in the immediate care of many patients with horrific injuries, which many modern day nurses will never have to deal with.

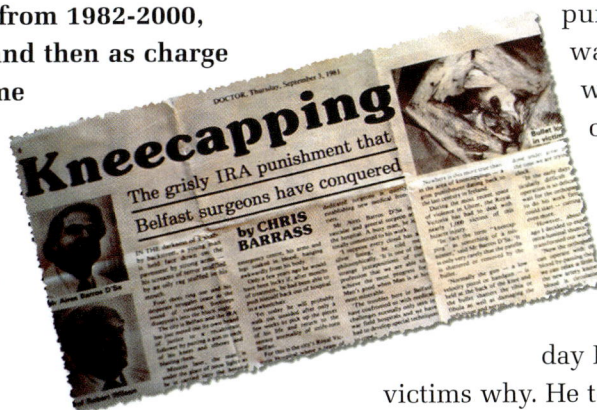

Tarring and feathering was one of the earliest forms of punishment used in the Troubles. Here tar was poured over the individual and a bag of feathers then applied, which would stick to the tar.

They were very difficult to clean, and we first came across them when we were working in the old City Hospital (before the Tower Block). I can remember a solvent called Tween 80 being used to remove the tar, but the easiest way was to take the person to a ward and let them soak in a bath to try to remove as much as possible before the application of the Tween 80. All in all, it was a very dirty job for the staff and highly traumatic for the victim.

Punishment beatings were very common and barbaric, resulting in multiple fractures. I have seen hands that had breeze-blocks dropped on them resulting in breakage of all the metacarpal bones.

Like the beating, punishment shootings happened almost on a daily basis. The victims were usually teenage men who had been 'summoned' to receive their punishment, which was usually a gunshot wound to the leg or legs.

I remember that these victims always wore more than one pair of trousers, so one day I asked one of the victims why. He told me that 'it was to slow down the speed of the bullet and decrease the amount of pain'!

When on night duty, some nights we would receive anywhere between three and six punishment shootings, and we would say that 'the circuit judge was out that night'! Some victims would have more than one gunshot wound, having been shot in both arms, knees and ankles. We called this 'an Ulster Fry'. Don't ask me why, as I think it was a phrase coined by the Ambulance Service.❞

A lucky escape...

"One night on night duty in Altnagelvin we were alerted to expect a young male with a gunshot wound to his knee.

We waited and waited and eventually the ambulance crew returned to base with no patient on board.

They told us that when they arrived at the scene the job hadn't been done and they were told to take a walk. After they heard the shot they returned to the scene and went on to assist the casualty. When they had driven some distance, in fact quite near the hospital, the casualty asked could he be taken to a local housing estate where his sister lived.

Enquiring after the wound, the ambulance staff were told that his assailants had missed and the bullet had gone through his jeans and had completely missed his leg.

After that, we were told, rules changed. It became compulsory to pull trouser legs above the knee before the punishment was delivered.**"**

Kneecapping in Craigavon

"I was a young 18 year old from the Republic of Ireland and began nurse training in Craigavon Area Hospital. While I was aware of religious discrimination, it was only during my training that I became aware of the extent of the Troubles and the depth of hatred and man's inhumanity to man.

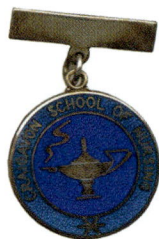

As a student I had nursed several young men who had been kneecapped and a few who had been beaten with baseball bats covered in six-inch nails. These left their victims with quite a number of puncture holes around legs and buttocks. Indeed I was surprised that a few of these young men took a kind of pride from this punishment. It seemed to provide a status as 'tough men' in their area.

During my surgical placement I nursed two men, one a policeman and the other a Republican, both of them were admitted with gunshot wounds from the same incident. Neither was seriously wounded as each was shot in the leg. What was surprising to me was the fact that both men were nursed in the same ward side-by-side. They talked in a friendly manner to each other. Indeed when one was in X-ray or physio, the other would purchase a newspaper or cigarettes for them when the shop came around each morning. Indeed if you didn't know, they could have been taken for friends or neighbours.

However, the difficulty was at visiting time when the families came. Each visitor glared angrily at the other patient and their friends and relatives, speaking loudly and negatively about the 'other side'. The curtains had to be drawn so that each wouldn't see the other. I asked the Republican patient why he had taken such a violent stance as he seemed to get along well with the policeman. He replied that his fight was against the British and those perceived to be maintaining British rule. He was shooting not at the person but at the ideology. He dismissed any human reaction, emotion or compassion. To me his perceived ideological stand seemed to dehumanise individuals and the people involved."

Eucalyptus oil

"As a student nurse I was on placement in the accident and emergency department of the Royal Victoria Hospital in 1976. One evening, when reporting for night duty, the sister in charge of the unit asked me if I had ever seen anyone who had been 'tarred and feathered'. When I said I hadn't, she handed me a plastic apron, a pair of gloves, several packets of gauze wipes and a bottle of eucalyptus oil and said 'Come with me'.

She brought me into a cubicle opposite her office where a young female patient was sitting on a trolley. Her hair had been 'cut' and her head, face and upper body were covered with tar and feathers. Sister proceeded to show me how to remove the coating and then left me to complete the task. It took me some time! I began by 'plucking' as many feathers as possible out of the tar and then started removing the tar itself. Getting the balance, between rubbing hard enough to remove the tar but gently enough so as not to remove the underlying skin, was an art.

I had heard on the news about people being 'tarred and feathered', but as a young student nurse from West of the Bann, seeing it in reality was something else. To this day, each time I smell eucalyptus oil, I think of that night in 1976."

A pool of tar and feathers

"It had been yet another busy day in casualty; I had been in the minor clinic all day and dealt with the usual stream of patients. Thankfully it had been a relatively normal day with no major incidents or serious cases arriving through the plastic doors.

I was excited as it was nearly 5pm, I was due off duty at 5.15pm and was looking forward to going out on a first date that night. Suddenly the doors flew open and down the corridor one could hear shouting and the sound of crying. When I looked out from the cubicle I saw a person, quite indistinguishable, covered in a black substance with feathers and other materials attached. It was a victim of 'tarring and feathering', a so-called punishment normally meted out to those whose behaviour had been deemed by some faceless group as unacceptable.

We rushed towards this screaming person and led her into a cubicle. The woman, who was hysterical, began flailing about, unsure of what was happening and worse still, what was going to happen. Eventually we calmed her and began the long, slow process of removing the tar and feathers.

Many deem this to be a minor injury, more a lesson in gross humiliation with little after effect. Not so. One is unsure of what lies beneath the tar as many victims of this crime are beaten before the final act; and tar, feathers and open wounds do not make for a happy combination. The physical injuries of course pale into insignificance when compared to the emotional damage, the impact of which can remain forever.

During the process we talked, slowly at first; in Belfast, silence reigned, permission to speak was often withheld, even if the person to whom you spoke wore a nurses' uniform. Eventually the physical cleansing was more or less complete; the emotional cleansing would take much longer.

We spoke of what her hair had been like before it was so roughly sheared, what her face had been like before the blows had rained down. We also spoke of her love for another, which had apparently brought this about. Frequently, the nurse in charge would put her head around the curtain and check how we were getting on. Unfortunately most of the tar and feathers were now adhered to my uniform, the patient sitting in a chair and I, on my knees on the ground. Both of us, surrounded by the debris of mulch, replied each time sister asked the question: 'Oh, we're fine.'

Physical cleansing complete, my patient was to be transferred to admissions for the night in order that her condition could be monitored. I brought her to the overnight bay, handed her over to my colleagues. As I was leaving she stood up and hugged me, thanking me for something I couldn't really hear.

My feelings welled up and I needed to go. I left and, walking towards Musson, I met a friend. 'Thought you were going on a big date tonight?' she said. I'd forgotten. Pity really, he seemed nice. But as it was our first date I had no contact details and I never saw him again – he probably thought I just stood him up. Why would he ever think I was standing in a pool of tar and feathers?

Next day I went to the sewing room to get another apron, the one from the previous evening had to be binned. 'What you young girls do with these uniforms I just don't know,' said the kindly woman in the sewing room. Indeed, what did I do with them? I seemed to go through an awful lot of aprons. I still have one of them. I take it out and look at it sometimes. I still see the stains of blood, tears and iodine. I put it away again as I don't like to go back there. Some stains just never came out. **"**

Major incidents 1969-1979

"Many nurses I know still get flashbacks of some of the horrific injuries they saw. Others find some memories too difficult to deal with; they cannot speak of them and have them deeply buried in their minds."

Mental Health Nurse

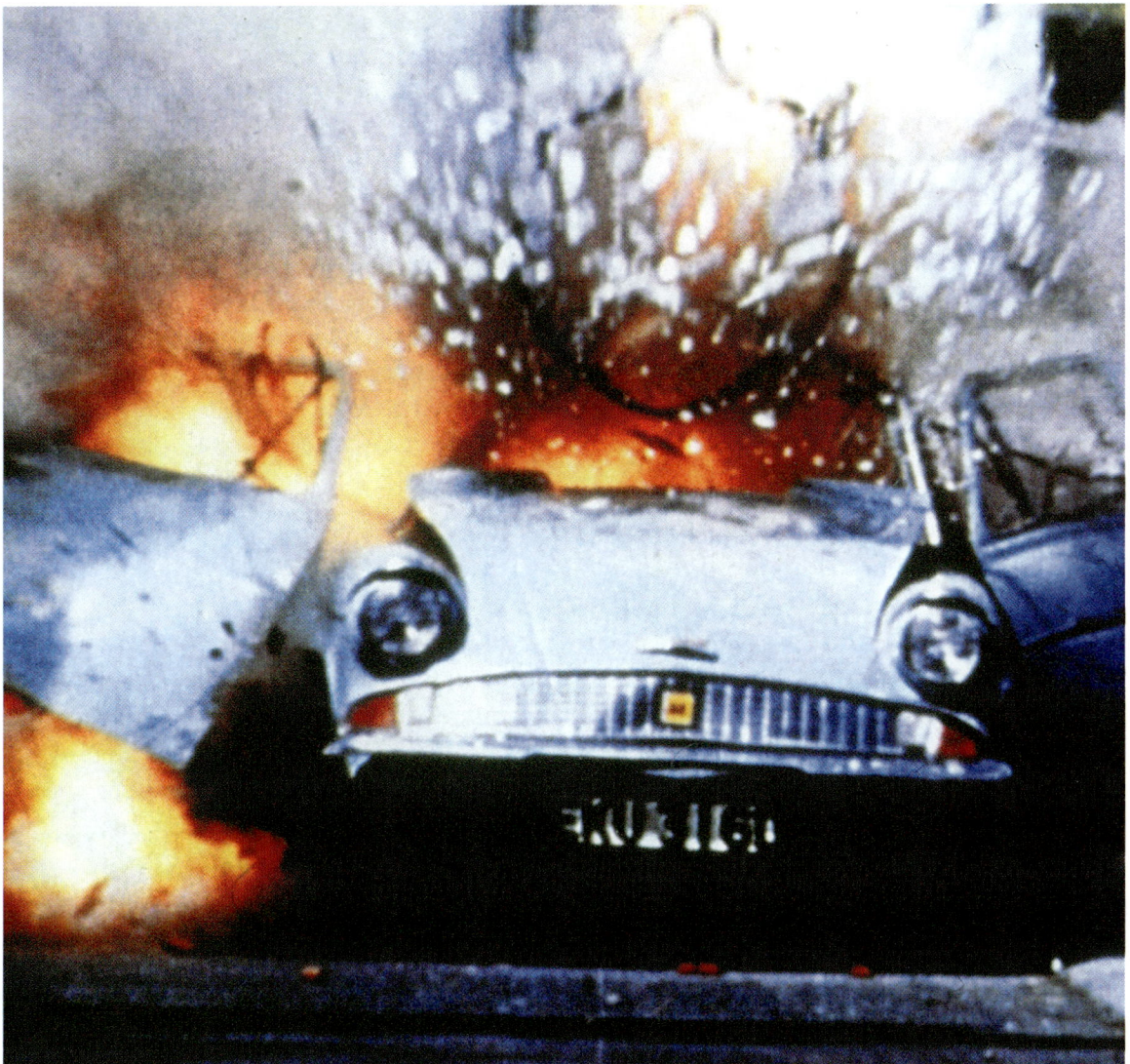

Exploding car bomb early 1970s

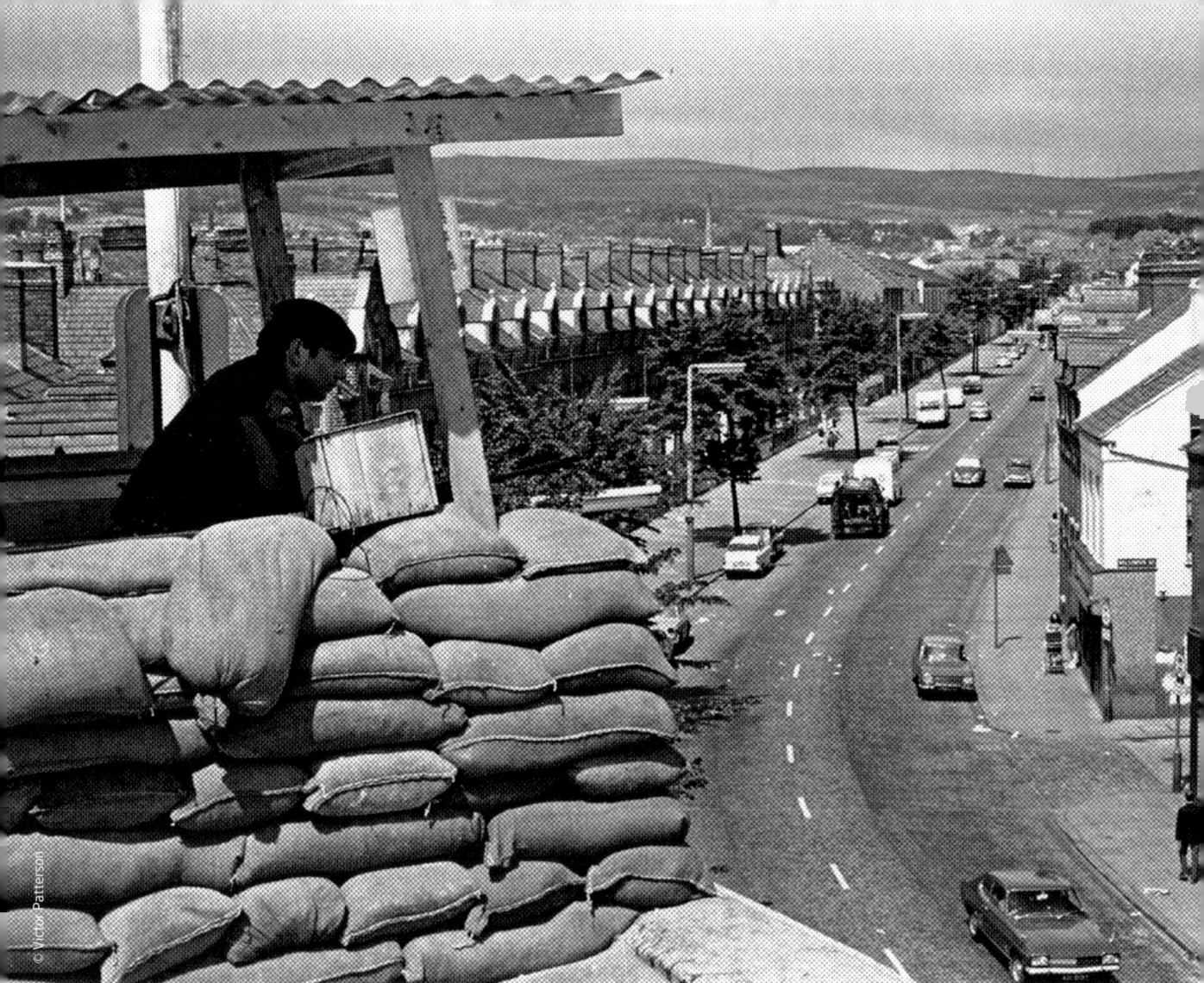

Soldier in lookout, Springfield Road, RUC Station 1971

The greatest number of lives were lost in 1972, mostly due to sustained bombing in towns across the province, particularly in Belfast and Derry/Londonderry. Most of the fatalities and injured in these incidents were civilians. Some of the stories recounted are from nurses who found themselves nursing casualties of their own age. Many found it especially distressing to nurse their contemporaries.

The Springfield Road Police
Station bomb
25 May 1971

A wake-up call

**❝I was a staff nurse, and later a sister,
in the accident and emergency unit at the
Royal Victoria Hospital, Belfast from April
1971 to December 1975. I was consequently
present for many of the major incidents.**

I arrived in casualty just as the rioting 'phase'
was beginning to give way to the bombing
campaign. This usually meant a decrease in
the number of incidents involving large
numbers of casualties with mostly minor
injuries, and an increase in admissions of
smaller numbers of casualties but with a
higher percentage of serious injuries.

One evening, shortly after I had joined the
staff, there was an explosion at Springfield
Road Police Station. The only serious
casualty was a soldier who was already dead
on arrival. He was 28 years old, married with
two children at home in England, and had
run back into the station when he heard
about the bomb to help move to safety some
local people who were there, ironically, to
complain about the army. He himself was the
last to leave and paid with his life. He lay on
the floor of the ambulance with his brain
tissue leaking all around him.

It was to be the first of many such
experiences during the next five years,
but it was the more memorable for being
the first one, and a wake-up call about the
reality of what was happening all around
me in Northern Ireland.❞

Act of bravery

**❝One night in May 1971, I had entered my
second year of training and was working
in ward 21, a neurosurgical ward with a
theatre attached. At about 8.15pm, I was
walking past the casualty department when
I heard an extremely loud blast. This was
not uncommon and I continued on my way.**

When I reached the ward, I was informed
that there had been a major explosion
outside the Springfield Road Police Station
and that a casualty was coming straight to
the ward.

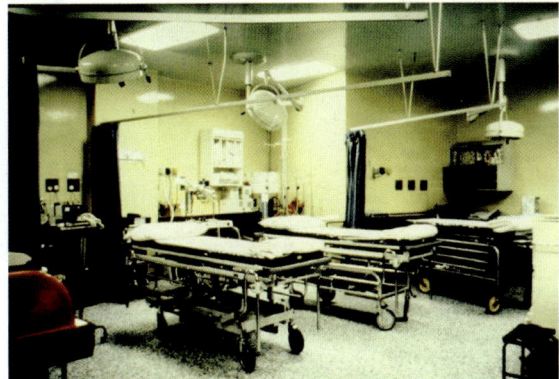

Resuscitation area, casualty, 1970s

The casualty arrived at approximately
8.45pm and was brought to an empty space
in a four-bed ward. I remember a number
of senior doctors and consultants putting
in an airway, erecting drips and lines,
and assessing the patient's injuries.
He had severe head injuries, was bleeding
profusely and was being transfused
with blood.

He had a drip in his left foot and my job
was to squeeze the bag of blood. As quickly
as I squeezed the bag, the blood was pouring

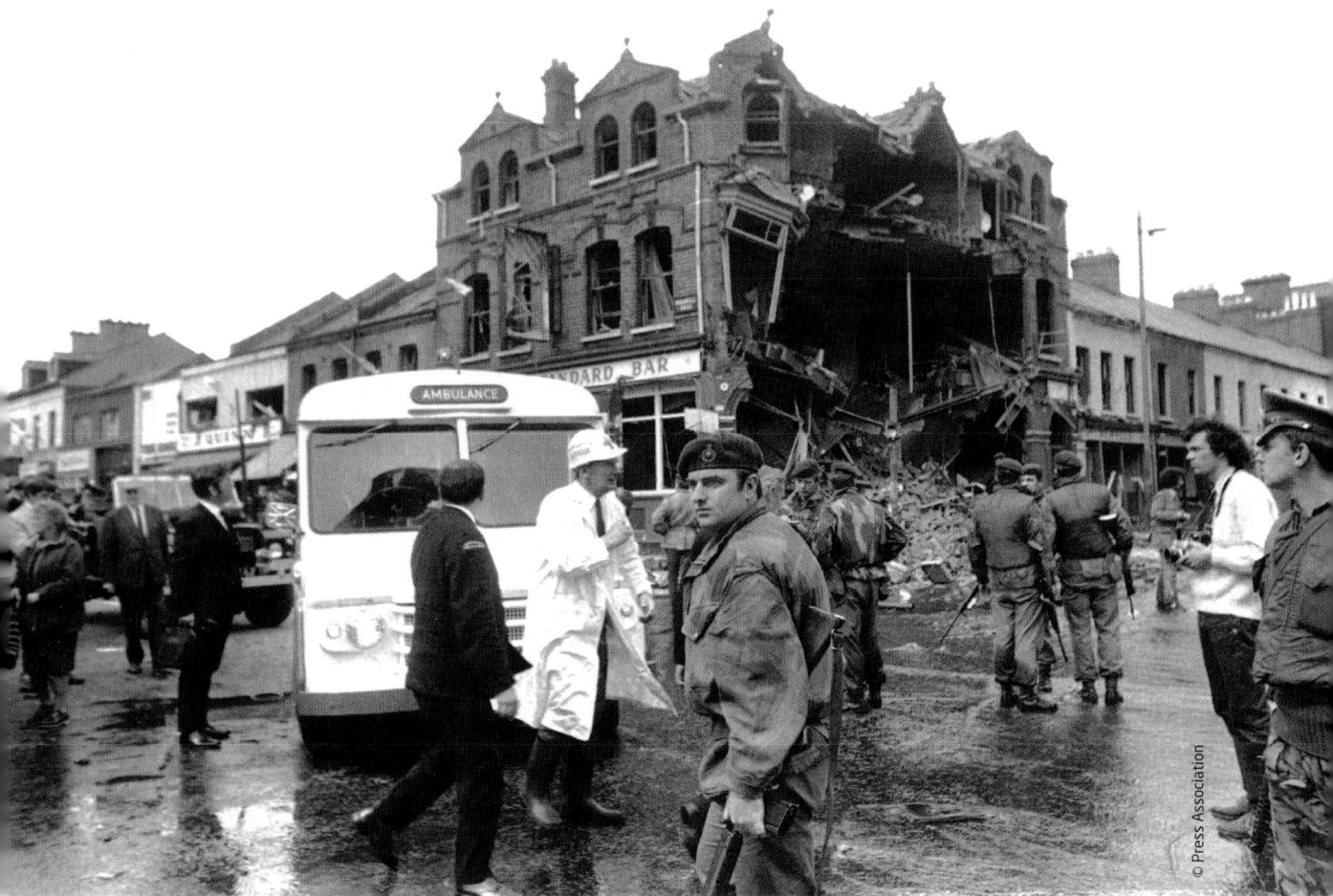
Another Shankill Road bomb, 1972

from his head. At approximately 10.45pm, two hours after admission, he was pronounced dead. With the help of another nurse, we proceeded to prepare the body for the mortuary. When the body was taken I cleaned the blood from the bed and floor and eventually had my first break at about 1.30am. I then continued the rest of my shift.

This young man was 28 years of age and a member of the British army who through his bravery had lost his life trying to save the lives of adults and children. He was posthumously awarded the George Cross.

I was only 18 when I had to deal with this situation. I can recall the whole event as if it were yesterday. How did I feel? Well, no one asked. In those days counselling was not something I was ever offered, indeed I do not even know if such services were available.

My way of dealing with such traumatic events was to have a cup of tea, a chat with friends, shed a few tears and just keep going. I believe that is the way most, if not all, of us coped with these traumatic events. The word 'stress' is not a word we were familiar with back in the 1970s.**

Internment
9 August 1971

"I was in charge of the casualty department on night duty when Internment began in the early hours of Monday morning. We had no warning before casualties began arriving on foot and in private cars. Within a very short time we were flooded with large numbers of people, some of whom were shouting hysterically and some of them verbally abusing staff.

Passions were running high, and at one point, a very well-known Member of Parliament went so far as to hit me. Casualty staff were often subjected to verbal abuse, but very occasionally it became physical.

When I went off duty later that morning and walked across to the hospital flats, everywhere I looked there were palls of black smoke all around the city. It was clear that we were on the verge of something very grave indeed. For the first time in my life, I believed that we could be about to embark on another war.

When I got up later that evening to go on duty, my flat-mate was listening to the local news which was recounting various incidents of shooting and announced that several people with gunshot wounds had been admitted to the RVH. I remember asking her to turn off the radio, which she was unwilling to do, not understanding that this was, in effect, my night report!

I then went on duty to a hectic night of activity during which we admitted 30 people with gunshot wounds. It was over 25 years before I could bear to listen to the Northern Ireland news again.**"**

Balmoral Furniture Company blast, Shankill Road
11 December 1971

"I was standing inside the Emergency entrance when an ambulance man ran in and thrust a bundle of rather grubby blankets into my arms. I couldn't understand why he was expecting me to dispose of what I thought was dirty laundry. I glanced down into the bundle and found myself looking into the face of a dead baby. The child's face had been rendered concave by the force of the blast and the features were barely recognisable."**

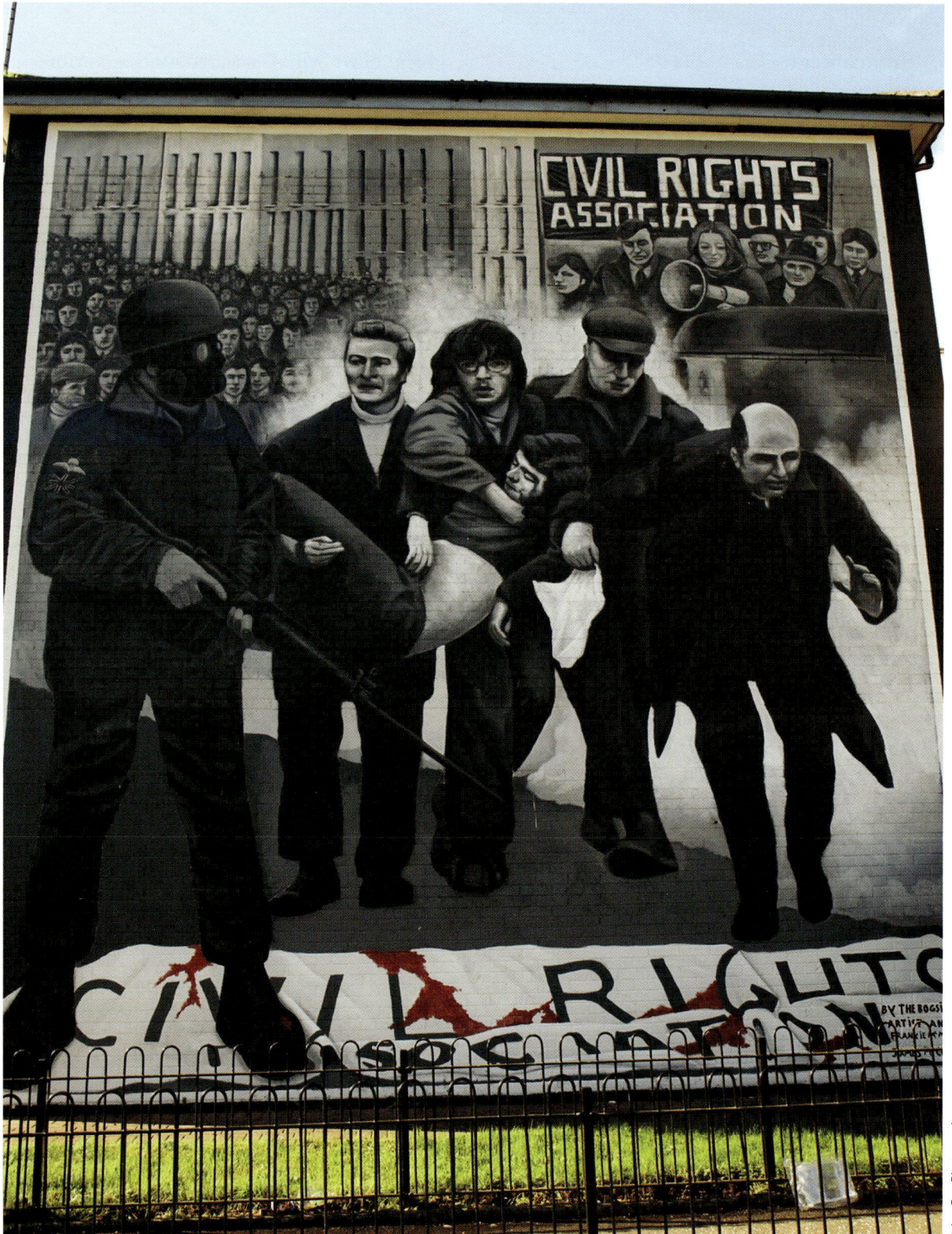

Bloody Sunday, Derry/Londonderry mural

Bloody Sunday
30 January 1972

Bloody Sunday remains among the most significant events in the Troubles of Northern Ireland, chiefly due to the fact that the shootings were carried out by the army and not paramilitaries, and in full public view. Twenty seven civil rights protesters were shot by the British army Parachute Regiment during a Northern Ireland Civil Rights Association march in Derry. Thirteen people died on the day.

This incident was contentious as the army maintained that they had been fired on first, this being denied by many witnesses. The findings of the Saville enquiry 2010 confirmed that the victims were unarmed civilians.

For nurses who worked in Altnagelvin Hospital, that day is well remembered and some are still haunted by flashbacks to sights witnessed.

Flashbacks and sleepless nights

❝Bloody Sunday is one of my most vivid memories. I was in a house in Rossville Street, Derry, watching the march when the shooting started. It seemed like an eternity until the gunfire stopped. I was scared and had a cold feeling in my chest coupled with a feeling of disbelief.

On looking out of the window I could see bodies lying unceremoniously on the deserted streets. My professional mind said 'go and cover them up' though my subconscious was saying 'don't go out there'. I took blankets from the house and, taking someone with me, I crossed the street cautiously and placed the blankets over several bodies. The silence was palpable with only some subdued sobbing. I shouted at one of the soldiers 'why did you do it?' but he gave no reaction.

Shortly after, I met up with one of the anaesthetists from Altnagelvin and we were asked to look at some of the wounded. We helped to place some people into ambulances and I joined one and went to report to the theatres in Altnagelvin where I was a staff nurse.

I went straight to work to help with the injured and worked all night. The atmosphere was very tense in theatres with remarks being made by several staff as to the rights and wrongs of what had happened. Sad but perhaps to be expected at that very difficult time.

That shift was one of the most chaotic nights I remember in theatre. But by the time we had lived through the Ballykelly and Enniskillen bombings, things were a lot more organised with the major emergency plan in place and working smoothly, even down to the pre-ordered refreshments.

No counselling was ever offered to me or my colleagues until after the Greysteel shootings, but by then I had learned to compartmentalise the events. However, after Bloody Sunday I had flashbacks and many sleepless nights about whether I had done enough to save people and what I would do in the future.

The injuries to patients' faces, necks and eyes are most prominent in my memory. I worked with outstanding facial/maxillary and ophthalmic surgeons. Seeing a bomb victim's face being scrubbed with a nailbrush to remove all the debris and the intricate internal and external fixations was just amazing. Years later I went to a world nursing conference in Vancouver and, during a lecture on gunshot and bomb damage to the face, I was proud when the lecturer, on learning I was from Northern Ireland, praised the knowledge he had gained from the surgeons who had worked in our war-torn times.

Many a planned operating list was interrupted by casualties of the Troubles. All theatre staff became adept at switching from hernias to gunshot wounds to the head, face, limbs or chest. Like all theatre sets, 'scenery' could be changed and within minutes instrumentation and surgeons were switched smoothly. We were top professionals within our fields.**"**

A horrific day

"I started nursing in Altnagelvin Hospital in September 1968 and completed training in 1971. I was 21 years old.

It was during this time that the Troubles started. We had not been trained in the care of gunshot wounds or blast injuries, but these were injuries that were to become commonplace for nursing and medical staff for many years to come. Sometimes these were a daily occurrence during my early years as a staff nurse at Altnagelvin A&E.

I was very aware that we were experiencing a vastly different climate to that which we had become accustomed.

During those first few months whilst I was on duty, a number of RUC men were shot and fatally wounded. There was nothing medicine could offer these men, but the need for identification meant I had to retrieve any personal effects which would help with this. I put my hand into the pocket of one man and removed some papers among which was a family photograph of beautiful children. I was so aware that these children would never see their dad again and I have to say that greatly disturbed me.

I didn't know if I could continue to work in an environment where these kinds of events would become a regular occurrence. However I did stay and witnessed many tragic events. I was on duty on Bloody Sunday – what a horrific day that was. It started as a fairly normal day. We were aware that there was a march but had no reason to believe that it would be any different to any other march.

There was no emergency plan as these were developed in later years. My fiancé had told me about the march and that he would be attending as he had a very keen interest in photography.

I remember taking a telephone call from a lady who said she was a theatre nurse and that a young male had been shot and we should expect him soon. We alerted senior surgical staff and set about getting IV fluids ready for his arrival. Time passed and no casualty arrived; this was an unusual delay.

Eventually the doors opened and I will never forget the pain, grief and terror that followed on that day.

Ambulance trolleys arrived; one after another, some with fatal injuries and some with severely injured young males and one female, who had all suffered gunshot wounds. The department was very small; two examination rooms, each with a changing cubicle about the size of a broom cupboard.

Relatives started turning up and searching for family members who were on the march. The thought of my fiancé crossed my mind. Was he going to arrive on a trolley wounded or worse? It seemed no one would have been safe that day.

Senior medical staff from all specialties arrived at the hospital and tried to establish some kind of order and organise theatre lists for surgical and orthopaedic theatres. After some time, order was restored to the department. All of the patients who had been wounded had been moved on to theatre where the medical and nursing staff worked through the night and well into the next day to provide the necessary care for all injured in this atrocity.

I only ever experienced similar distress on two other occasions. One was at the Hallowe'en night shootings at the Rising Sun bar in Greysteel, and the second was the Omagh bomb. There was a real sense of anger, distress, confusion, grief and sense of loss in all three events.

I spent 38 years working in A&E, I loved my work, met beautiful people, both patients and staff, made many lifelong friends and we still meet regularly. We worked through some very difficult times and there was no counselling in those days. We counselled each other and buried our thoughts if they were too difficult to dwell on. I'm sure that these events have left a mark on all the staff who worked through these times.

I had a great working life despite the many tragedies which we had to witness. It was a privilege to have been part of it. "

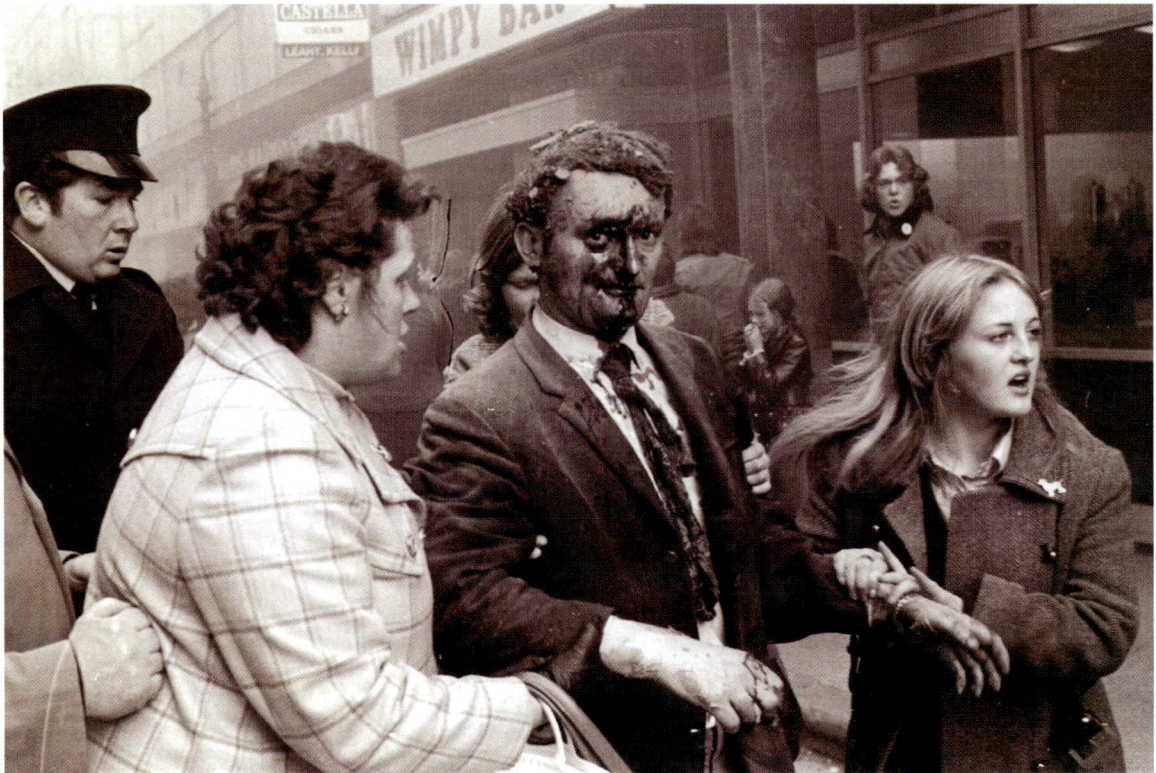

Abercorn bombing 1972 – more than 130 people were hurt

The Abercorn Restaurant Bomb
4 March 1972

"One of the things which made this explosion so traumatic for staff members was that the Abercorn Restaurant was one of our favourite venues for coffee with friends and we knew that any one of us could have been there that day."

RVH Staff Nurse

The Abercorn Restaurant bombing was an attack that took place in a crowded city centre restaurant and bar in Belfast. The city was full of Saturday shoppers and the Abercorn was a popular restaurant on Castle Lane, a narrow street at the back entrance to many of the high street shops on Royal Avenue.

The bomb exploded at 4.30pm claiming the lives of two young women and injuring more than 130 people.

Many casualties sustained life-threatening and life-changing injuries., including the loss of limbs and eyes, eardrums were burst, lungs rattled causing respiratory blast damage. Flying debris as large as table legs and as fine as shards of glass were embedded in over 100 casualties. Eleven shattered limbs were amputated; two sisters lost five limbs between them. Survivors still live with their physical and emotional injuries.

A staff nurse on duty in the Royal Victoria Hospital casualty recalls it as one of her darkest days…

"I was in charge of casualty that Saturday afternoon and we thought it unusually quiet for a week-end 'take-in', which was just as well because we were not over-staffed that day. I just happened to ring up ambulance control to find out why they hadn't collected a couple of patients from our observation ward and was told that they didn't have time because they were dealing with a 'massive' bomb in town and that there were 'probably over 300 casualties'.

It was unusual for Ambulance Control not to warn us of a major emergency ahead of admission, but they had forgotten in all the panic. We were left with insufficient time to prepare for the worst explosion in terms of casualties that we'd ever had.

My personal memory is being on the phone to ask nursing administration for help while the rest of the staff desperately tried to clear the cubicles of all non-emergencies, against a backdrop of the noise of the approaching ambulances coming ever nearer. When they stopped outside casualty, they usually switched off the klaxons because the sound would be further exaggerated under the covered entrance. On this occasion, the drivers hadn't remembered to do this, another sure sign of panic, with the result that the collective noise of several ambulances queuing up was deafening.

In spite of this, the screams of the casualties inside the ambulances could be heard above this noise. At the same time I was hearing a Nursing Officer telling me over the phone that she was unable to send me any help. That moment has stayed with me over the years as probably the worst of many bad experiences during that period.

What made this explosion so traumatic for staff members was that the Abercorn Restaurant was one of our favourite venues for coffee with friends, and we knew that any one of us could have been there on that day. As it happened one of our own casualty radiographers, who had been on duty that morning, had gone there on her afternoon off. The next time I saw her, I was holding her body pieces in a number of plastic bags. Her father was an anaesthetist in the hospital and had been called in for duty and was working in theatre.

Needless to say, there was no such thing as counselling for nurses or anyone else in those days. I wasn't really aware of any psychological effects until I went into a butcher's shop a few days later. When I looked at all that raw meat laid out in the window, I had to leave the shop immediately. It was some time before I could look at meat again.

Many years later, while struggling with a problem in statistical analysis during my degree studies, I approached a maths teacher who had been recommended by a friend. I noticed that she had a pronounced limp and asked her if she had had an accident. She replied that she had lost a leg during the Abercorn explosion more than 16 years before. It was good to know that at least some of the many casualties we had cared for on that dreadful day had survived and gone on to lead something approaching a normal life."

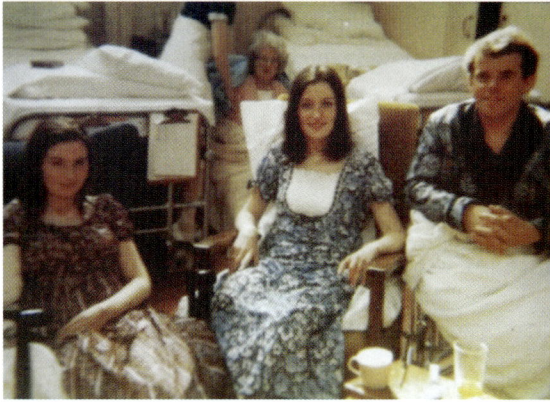
Abercorn bomb casualties, including McNern sisters and Jimmy Stewart

McNern sisters

I SHOULD LIKE, through your paper, to express my gratitude to the staff of the Royal Victoria Hospital and Musgrave Park Hospital for their devoted attention to my two daughters, Rosaleen and Jennifer, during the past 12 months.

I wish to thank especially the surgeons, the staff of the Respiratory and Intensive Care Unit and Ward 17 of the "Royal," also all those involved in their wellbeing whilst they were patients in Withers Block and the Limb-fitting Centre of Musgrave Park Hospital.

Thank you also to the ambulance men for their prompt and sympathetic attention and my wonderful neighbours and friends, old and new, without whose support and kindness I could never have coped.

(Mrs.) TERESA McNERN, 63 Manor Street, Belfast 14.

Abercorn bomb 1972 – aftermath

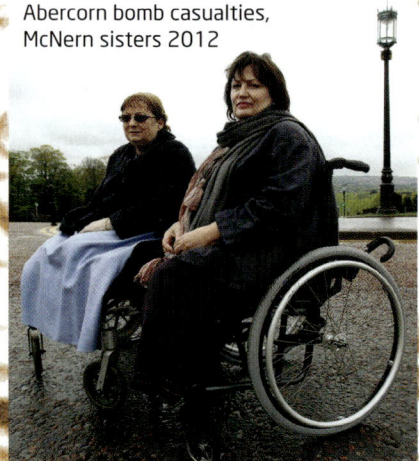
Abercorn bomb casualties, McNern sisters 2012

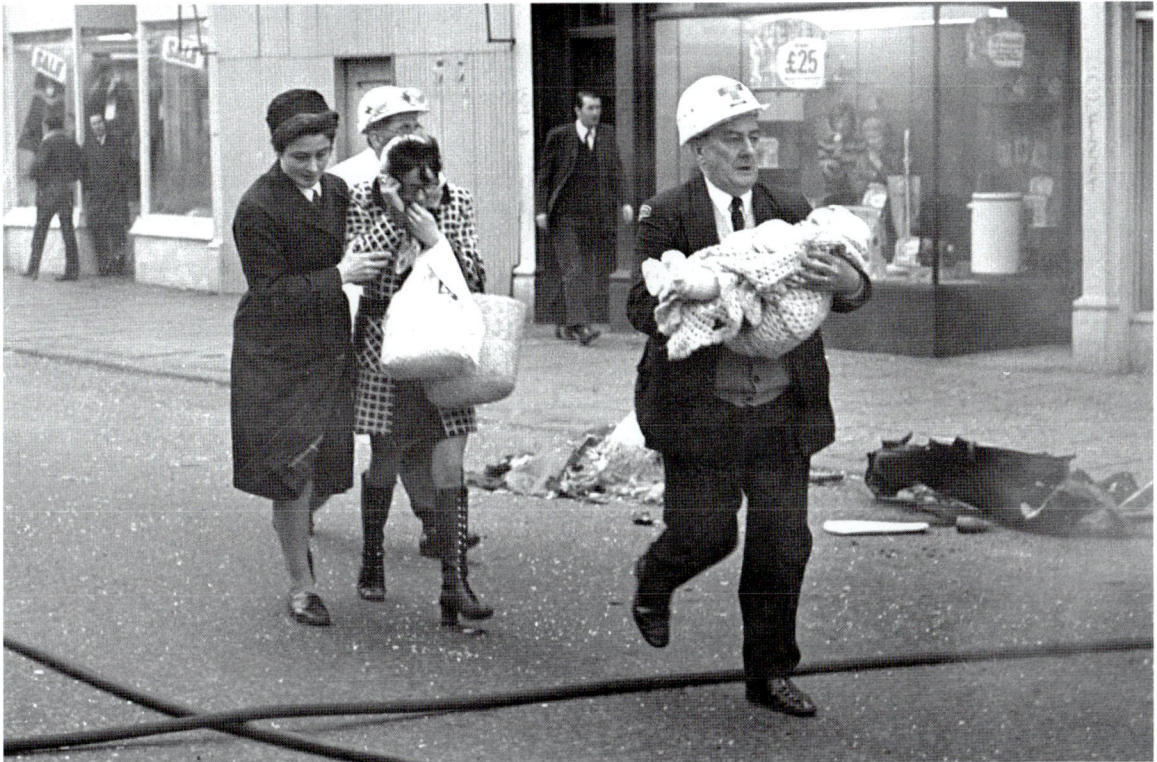

© Victor Patterson

Bloody Friday – Bradbury Place car bomb, Belfast 1972

Bloody Friday
21 July 1972

On this afternoon, 22 bombs exploded across Belfast in the space of 75 minutes. Security forces had to manage hoax calls as well as explosions. Nine people were killed; the youngest was 14 years old. Of the 130 injured, many were maimed for life.

The young boy

A casualty staff nurse remembers that day...

❝ Ambulance crews normally transported the bodies of the dead directly to the mortuary, only stopping en route at casualty for formal certification. But where large numbers of casualties were involved, they often had to return immediately to the scene of the explosion and so would leave the bodies with us for disposal. This meant that we had to set up a makeshift mortuary and we used a room at the back of the department for this purpose.

On Bloody Friday a young boy was brought in dead, and soon after a man arrived looking for his son. His description fitted that of the dead child and, while I warned him that we could not be certain, I was obliged to take him to see the body.

When he saw the dead boy he realised that he was not his son, but his reaction was shocking. Instead of being relieved and thankful, he became furiously angry and began to accuse me of having given him a terrible and unnecessary fright. There seemed to be no sense of grateful relief that his own son was now probably safe, somewhere – or pity for the family of the dead boy before him.

In A&E, we were used to receiving rather less patient appreciation than ward staff who had more long-term contact. However that particular reaction took even the security man by surprise."

Feeling helpless

A student nurse recalls...

"I was working on that afternoon in ward 26 – dermatology. I can remember it was a lovely afternoon. I must have been out on the balcony with patients when we heard loud explosions. We could see smoke appearing in the sky over the city.

Very quickly after this there was the sound of sirens all going at the same time. Before these sounds faded there was the new noise of police and army vehicles pulling into the hospital grounds. Their doors were open and it looked from a distance as if injured people were in the back of these Land Rovers en route to casualty.

Porters were arriving up into the ward taking any equipment that was not in use and telling us that bombs had gone off in Belfast with many people injured, some probably dead.

Patients were upset as they didn't know if someone they loved was caught up in this. You must remember this was before mobile phones so communication was therefore difficult. We did our routine tasks, made cups of tea for distressed patients and generally tried to do anything that we could do to assist, even though we felt quite helpless in the situation."

A holiday feeling...

"The child health clinic was busy. The buzz of chatter, children playing, and the noise of teacups. The room was full of mothers waiting for their children's developmental screening with us, the health visitors. A lovely Friday afternoon in July with almost a holiday feeling.

The bomb went off at 3pm. A collective intake of breath, the instinctive gathering of wee ones to their mothers. The smoke drifting in the clear sky. Nervous laughter hastily stopped. All had been here before. How big was the bomb, how near, what did it mean?

The bombs continued to explode… Two… Three… Four… Five… panic set in. We all knew this meant terror and destruction on a large scale. Mothers wanted to get home to the phone, to family, to the safety of their own place. As they left with crying children, apologising to us for going, the bombs continued to echo across the city.

Six… Seven… Eight… Nine… Ten… Who could imagine there would be 22 in total?

Who could imagine such cruelty? Who could conceive of such indiscriminate disregard for human life? Who could plan and direct such destruction on a lovely July day?

The rest of that day in the Royal, horror and disbelief at the sights and sounds of distraught relatives, the clatter of trolleys, frantic cries for help to overstretched medics and nurses… and still they came. What to do, how to help? Feelings of unreality, anger and then, later, an almost primeval desire for revenge.

I WISHED THEY COULD SEE WHAT THEY HAD DONE.

The trolley, lined with rows of plastic bags containing the remnants of lives and hopes and dreams. Guarding a trolley, receiving more and more bags, protecting and covering with towels and sheets in an attempt to bring a little dignity to a nightmare scene. A long night, filled with violent death, and inconsolable grief.

The epitome of horror.

Monday morning back in the clinic, three days after Bloody Friday. One mother lost her husband, blown up at the bus station coming home from work, identified only by his hand. That big coffin, for one hand.

Fractured lives.**"**

Claudy Village Bombing
31 July 1972

Three car bombs exploded mid-morning in the centre of the town of Claudy in County Derry/Londonderry, killing nine people. The explosions took place without warning, as the bombers' attempted warning was delayed by out-of-order telephones due to a previous bombing at the exchanges.

The attack killed six people immediately, with three later dying from their injuries. A young girl and two teenage boys were among the dead. A retired nurse from Altnagelvin Hospital was also killed.

A night nurse recalls...

❝I was working at Altnagelvin Hospital. I was in the operating theatre doing two nights per week. At that time I was living about five miles from Claudy.

On 31 July the village was bombed. It was a very tense time being the morning of 'Operation Motorman' when the army were moving into the Bogside to take over no-go areas. It was after 10am when my husband, who was working in Claudy, phoned to say that a bomb had exploded killing six people. One of them was a retired ward sister from the hospital.

That call was the first news that we heard of the bombs in Claudy. He had phoned when he was almost at the hospital from the first phone he found still working. The IRA had bombed the Feeny and Claudy phone exchanges the previous weekend. We were one of the few who had been given an emergency number.

My husband said that he, like others, ran to the village, not realising that there were two other car bombs about to explode. I rang the operating theatres explaining the situation asking that they contact A&E, as my husband and others were bringing in casualties.

I then went into theatre and everywhere I went I met neighbours and colleagues concerned that their families were caught up in the bombs. The village was blocked off and people were diverted up back roads. I only saw the carnage on my way home at 2am. I hardly recognised the village. In this atrocity there were nine people killed; five Protestants and four Catholics.❞

Travel, transport and telephones

" The commitment of staff getting to work throughout the civil unrest cannot be overemphasised. I remember a nurse was in a bus, which was hijacked and burnt. She went home and drove herself into work, uncertain of what might confront her on the way."

Senior Nurse

Falls Road demonstration outside Royal Victoria Hospital

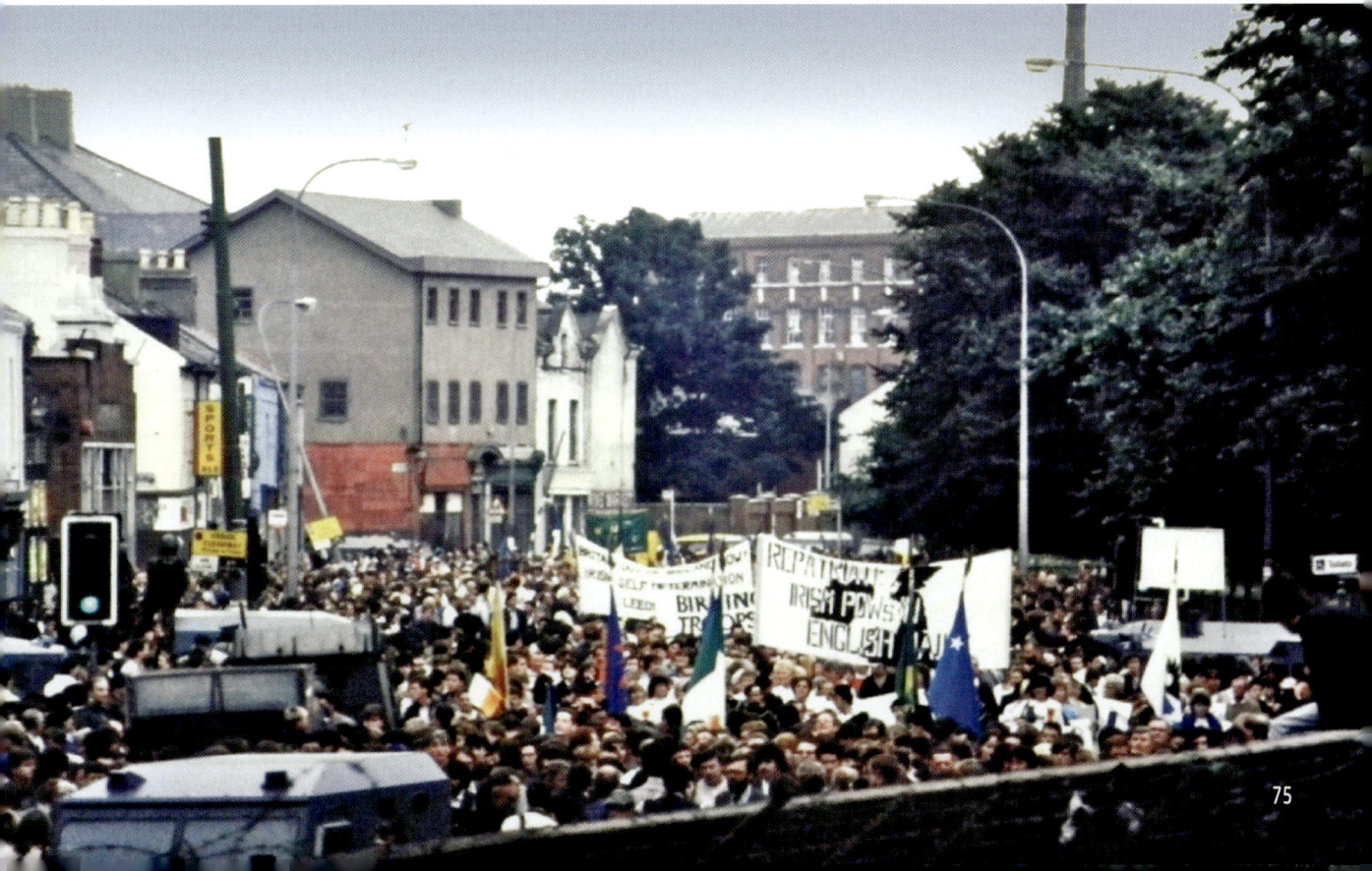

Many stories tell of difficulties in getting to and from work, even for those who lived close by. Few nurses owned a car and so relied on public transport. Some cycled. Buses were routinely withdrawn whenever violence erupted as they were frequently hijacked and used as barricades. Taxi drivers felt exposed if they drove outside their normal routes or if their taxi name indicated "which side" they were from. Nurses who lived a distance from their place of work often faced a long walk, and many were caught in crossfire. But regardless of all these obstacles, nurses still arrived at work.

"How they get here on time, no excuses, they're here."
Hospital Consultant MPH

"They have been getting to work for the past seven years... All grades are wonderful. They walk, use any means, never let us down, absenteeism is lower than any hospital in England."
Matron RVH (1976)

"Travel to and from the hospital was a major concern for many staff, but I do not remember a time when there was not a full complement of staff. Anxiety about getting home in the morning through wrecks of burned out cars to get children ready for school was a reality for staff living in West Belfast."
Sister RMH

There were occasions when transfer of patients between hospitals could be adventurous as well. The ambulances of the 1960s and 1970s did not contain today's sophisticated equipment. One nurse remembered travelling with a patient from Altnagelvin Hospital to Belfast. The route was not direct; the ambulance had to drive through towns that had a provincial hospital should medical help be required if the patient's condition deteriorated. On occasions nurses accompanied patients being transferred by army helicopter to hospital when urgent treatment was required.

For community nurses driving around certain districts was challenging. Nurses told of being stopped by masked men as they attempted to get through barricades. Others described the difficulty of identifying streets when all the street names had been removed or blacked out. Many were glad to wear a recognisable uniform.

During these early years of the Troubles many nurses did not have access to a telephone. Off duty nurses usually contacted their hospital to offer help when they heard of a major incident and media alerts were broadcast requesting staff to return to work. One nurse recalled how, following a serious explosion, she was collected, with no notice, by ambulance and brought to assist in theatre.

The following stories relate to various forms of travel and transport, including by foot, car, ambulance or air.

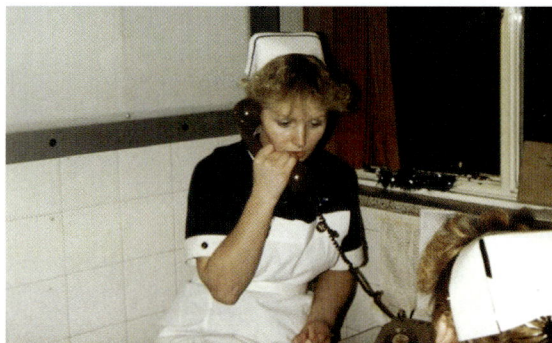

Altnagelvin Nurse on telephone 1970s

A new day

I walk along the Grosvenor Road in the cold grey dawn.
Another night of rioting and violence and death has passed.
When will they ever learn to live and let live?

My train from home was late.
Another bomb scare on the line.
And now there are no buses. And so I walk.

There are soldiers all along the road, armed with guns;
Stationed at corners in twos and threes.
They look at my case and stop me.
"Where are you going?" they say.
"I'm a RVH nurse going back on duty" I say,
And they let me through.

A solitary bread van crawls along the stone-strewn thoroughfare,
And furtive housewives hasten out to purchase of its wares.

I've reached my destination now.
Outside its red brick walls army jeeps and trucks are parked.
More questions, more checks:
My little case survives another search!

At last!
I step inside the thick, black, wrought-iron gates,
And feel security envelop me.

I'm back.
It's a new day!
Home and days off seem a million miles away.
For yet another while, we have a tense uneasy peace.
Tonight most likely, they will do it all again.

Vera E Poots (née Hunniford)

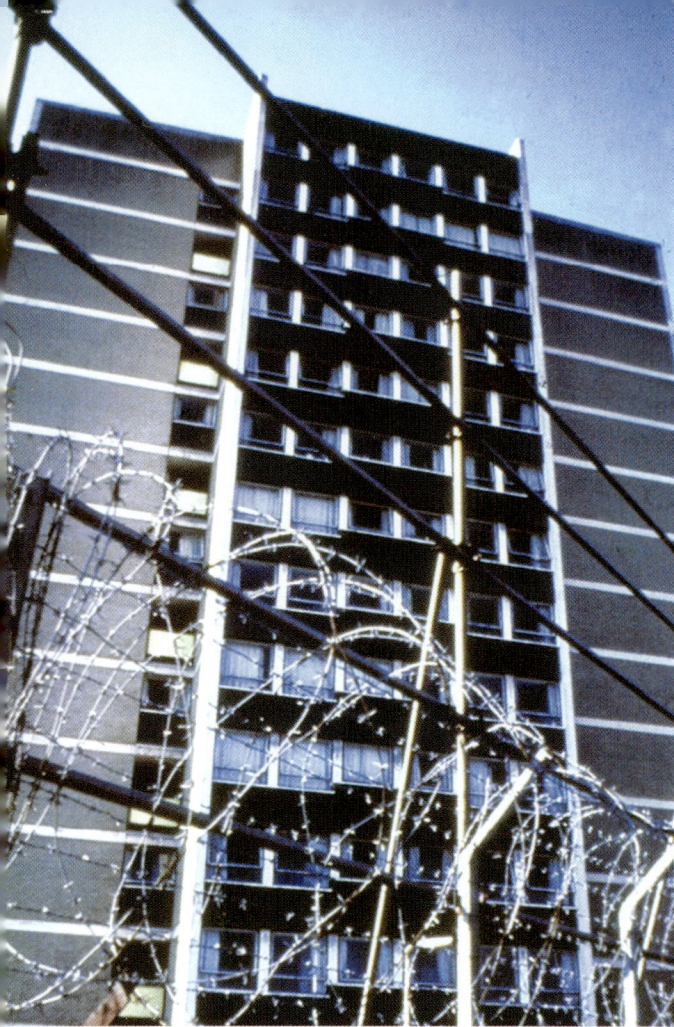
Broadway Towers

Living at the Towers

"I moved into the Towers beside the Royal Victoria Hospital (RVH) in 1969 and lived there for 20 years. All branches of medical, nursing and student staff were accommodated there. We overlooked Celtic Park Greyhound Stadium and the Maguire & Patterson match factory. It was convenient for the hospital but at times a very difficult place to live, with bomb scares, hijacking, burning of buses and taxis taking place over many years.

The Hospital Secretary lived on the site when he was 'on call'. He contacted us when we had to evacuate the buildings, which mostly occurred at night. There was never much time to gather up one's treasures, but some folk did! One never knew whether to go to bed early before the shooting started or stay up late in the hope that things might settle down. For a long time I always kept a pair of trousers and sweater by my bed at the ready. It did feel a bit unreal next morning when everyone was going about their business as normal.

On one occasion I did get an early morning call at 5am. It was from the police, asking if I was the owner of a silver Metro? When I said 'Yes, where is it?', I was informed that it was at Divis flats, having been stolen and used by joyriders, and would I come and identify it? Fortunately it was daylight. A friend accompanied me to the police station. We were taken in a Land Rover to my car. It was badly damaged. The police asked me to open the door as they watched from a distance, in case it was booby-trapped. I wished afterwards that the car had been irreparable.

As well as living with unrest in the surrounding area whilst working, life outside work was also difficult. It was not safe to walk around or drive after dark, so one was unable to attend church, visit friends or have many outside interests. We were fortunate to have a mini-supermarket on site to buy essentials.

One afternoon I was walking over to the Towers after my shift. It was a lovely sunny day and all was quiet, but then I heard this 'whizzing' noise. It sounded very close. When I met one of the hospital security men and asked him 'What was that?', his answer was: 'When you don't hear it you need to worry!' A shot had been fired and the noise was the bullet passing me, not very high above my head.

On another occasion a senior colleague of mine in the eye and ear clinic had changed her off-duty to cover the evening shift. When she returned to her flat about 9pm, she found a bullet had come through her window, so God was taking care of her too.

My father kept a very close ear to the Radio Ulster news bulletins. One evening I had just returned from the clinic at about 9pm. My phone rang. It was dad to ask if I was alright? Apparently a bomb had gone off outside the RVH during the day. He didn't believe me when I said I hadn't heard it and was about to listen to the 9pm news. Once one was on duty you got on with what needed to be done and were not always aware what was going on outside. There were always patients to care for and reassure. **"**

Disturbed nights

Another nurse remembers…

"I worked in the Royal Victoria Hospital throughout the years of the Troubles. For 20 of those years I lived in the Towers. Situated at Broadway, adjacent to the M1, this was one of three buildings which bordered two communities and were frequently the location of riots and gunfights between nationalists and loyalists.

In 1969 it was still possible to access the flat roof of the 12/13-storey buildings. This gave excellent views over the surrounding areas. When rioting peaked at the start of the Troubles on the night of 14 August 1969, I watched from this point as fires were lit and barricades were erected. Later this area was 'out of bounds' as an army observation post was established on the flat roof of one building.

Life was anything but quiet. On many occasions, I saw 'tracer' bullets as I looked over the grounds of what was then Celtic Park. Sometimes it was hard to distinguish whether gunshots or explosions were the television or activity in the surrounding area. Some colleagues had bullets fired into their flats. Fortunately I was not to experience this problem. Disturbed nights did happen, but more often than not, life went on as normal for residents. **"**

The Sunday Post

JUNE 28, 1981   No. 3956   Price 16p (Eire 22p)

Morning Special

BULLETS FLY IN HOSPITAL WARD

NURSES CAUGHT IN BATTLE TERROR

BELFAST TELEGRAPH REPORTERS 27.7.12

NURSES from the Royal Victoria Hospital described

Bullets hit nurses' home

Irish news 9.7.16

A Belfast nurses' home was hit by eight bullets in an attack thought to have been meant for an Army post at Broadway, just off the M1, last night.

Some windows in Victoria Towers were broken, but no casualties were reported. About 100 nurses live in the flats complex.

In Dungannon, a parcel

Nurses escape as shots hit home

Belf. Newsletter, 9.7.16

Terrorists bullets fired at the Army base at Broadway, West Belfast, last night, went wide and broke windows and struck walls in the nearby Victoria Towers Nurses Home.

None of the nurses was injured although some were later suffering from shock.

Eight shots were fired at the Army post at 9-30 p.m. but security forces said that none of the bullets hit their intended target and none of the personnel was injured.

One of the residents in the Nurses Home said: "We were having a quiet evening when we heard the bullets striking the walls and smashing windows. It was a nasty experience.

"For a moment we thought our building was the target but then we realised that the raiders had been firing at the Army post."

A bullet through my pillow

"My story began when my 15-year-old brother wanted to come to Belfast. He stayed with me in the Towers. On one particular night, the shooting erupted again. He was so excited by all of this. He opened the curtains and, unbeknownst to me, the window, so he could hear the bullets.

Instinctively I jumped out of bed and pushed him onto the bathroom floor. Suddenly there was a 'swish' followed by a loud blast inside my bedroom. As the shooting continued, I peeped out and could see dust and mortar and then a large hole in my wall just at my pillow. The pillow was in smithereens.

We went out into the communal corridor where my friends were sheltering on the floor. We grabbed duvets and joined them. The following day, army personnel arrived and removed the bullet lodged in the wall. I made my brother go home.

I went on duty that evening at 10pm and in the theatre block there were several squaddies positioned with their guns at the ready. This was a regular occurrence. Prisoners who had fought in jail were brought to us under armed guard.

My best friend was on holiday in Spain at the time and she bought an English newspaper. It included a short piece on how there had been another gun battle at the Royal Victoria Hospital and a nurse had had a bullet shot through her window. How my news had travelled!**"**

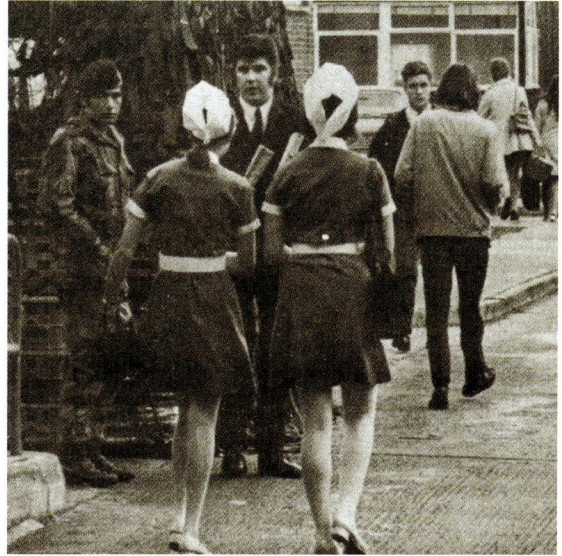

Student nurses and army, 1972

Student nurses' transport

"Coming on duty in October 1969 as student nurses returning to the Royal Belfast Hospital for Sick Children, four of us travelled back to Belfast on a Sunday night.

We left the train at the old Great Victoria Street Station and walked onto Sandy Row. Here we were met by paramilitaries wearing balaclavas who approached us and asked where we were going. We replied we were nurses returning to the hospital. Their response was 'you are doing a good job, on you go'. From there we walked up the Falls Road. Here we were met by more paramilitaries who asked the same question and also told us we were doing a good job and allowed us further up the Falls Road.

At the time we were more interested in what we had done over the weekend than what all this fuss was about.**"**

Hitchhiking home

"Many nurses thumbed lifts home in the early 1970s. I remember one Sunday afternoon by the Balmoral roundabout at the motorway, thumbing with my friend who was from Cookstown. Along came a big army lorry. It stopped and in jumped Eileen and I. Crazy or what?

We got a lift right into the square in Coalisland beside the police station. Out the pair of us jumped thankful to be home. Can you imagine that a few years on? We were innocent and oblivious to the danger that we could have been in. Coalisland was an IRA stronghold where many police and UDR men lost their lives. It was a different world with few rules and regulations back then."

Playing at the barricades

A theatre nurse recalls one journey to work that became a lasting memory…

"There was the difficulty of getting from home to work. Unofficial street barricades would be built at short notice, when local residents felt threatened or wished to show authority. A knowledge of different routes was essential. One nurse, new to Northern Ireland and with a poor sense of direction, was often in bother when trying to negotiate unfamiliar routes. No mobile phones then!

At 7.30am I came to a barricade where six or seven men told me I could not pass. I explained I was a nurse on my way to the Royal Victoria Hospital. They consulted each other for a minute then one came forward telling me that a little lad had been playing at the barricade. I did not ask why he was doing this at that time of the morning. He had fallen, and, using a colloquial term, described where he was cut (his privates). 'Would I look and advise?' He brought a lad of four or five years, who was persuaded to show the nurse the sore place. It was not a deep cut, but must have been hurting. I thought in case of infection or problems later, he should be seen at hospital. The offer to take him was gladly accepted.

We arrived by various side-streets and parted with thanks and good wishes to each other. Those macho men had shown their caring side. That wee frightened lad would be aged about 40 years now. I never pass that street without remembering him. I do hope his life has been happy and more peaceful than his early years."

Adventurous journeys to work at the Royal 1971-1973

"Whilst working as a staff nurse and junior sister at the Royal Victoria Hospital between 1971 and 1973, I lived in a suburb of North Belfast, close to the County Antrim countryside.

Going home by car at about 9pm could prove a challenge. First, it was wise to phone the ambulance station to find out which of the three possible routes from the hospital was likely to be the safest that night. Their advice would vary from night to night depending on the level of rioting, shooting and car hijacking going on around a particular main road. One night I remember weaving my way down the Grosvenor Road towards the city centre, avoiding cars that had been set alight and masked gunmen trying to hijack my car. I was driving on full headlights as all the street lighting had been shot out.

Another night I had to get from my ward to the car park, adjacent to the Dental School building. In the dark evenings this car park was floodlit. One evening as I ran to the car I remember thinking: 'Am I a sitting duck or a ballerina in the spotlight here?' There were a number of snipers with high velocity rifles situated on the top of the Dental School building. Many bursts of that 'ping-ping' sound rent the air as shots were fired towards the Grosvenor Road in Belfast. The gunmen could not have failed to see me, so perhaps my nurse's uniform saved me. Home that night was even sweeter than usual, even if my pulse rate was barely back to normal.

One light evening, cutting down a side-street by car, off the Grosvenor Road, I came across a young woman tied to a lamppost. Her head was shaven and she had been tarred and feathered. A small crowd were standing further down the narrow street. This type of punishment was meted out to women and men who were perceived by their local community to have acted against that particular society's norms.

Having seen this, what could I do to help? It was much too dangerous to stop and try to help directly, so I drove on until I came across some soldiers in an armoured personnel carrier (vehicles known as Pigs) which I flagged down.

I shouted up to the soldiers and asked them to rescue the woman, having pointed out the general direction that they should go.

I never knew what happened to that woman but I have always hoped that it was possible for her to be reintegrated into her community and not to have to flee to another country to ensure her safety.

On February 7 1973 the United Loyalist Council ordered a one-day strike throughout Ulster. I was due on an early duty that day and it was usual to travel in one's nurse's uniform at that time, in an attempt to enhance your personal security whilst travelling. Approaching the lower Falls Road at about 7.30am, I was stopped at an illegal roadblock by men carrying automatic machine guns and wearing balaclavas.

It was always wise to stop at these roadblocks, but I do remember having a heated discussion with these masked men. I asked who would be there to care for the sick and injured, including perhaps their friends and relatives, if they did not let me go to work. That did the trick and I was 'allowed' to proceed. I was, however, cross at the men's attempts to intimidate me and make me return home against my will. 🙶

The yellow suitcase

"I worked in the Royal Victoria Hospital as a nursing assistant for two months before starting my nurse training at the end of August 1975. I had been off for the weekend and my father was taking me back on the Sunday night. It was like a family outing as my brother and mother were with us too.

We were later than planned arriving in Belfast as we had a puncture on the way. Father drove the usual route by Ligoniel, down the Crumlin Road, Woodvale and Shankill and across Ainsworth Avenue to the Springfield Road [these were areas of intense civil unrest]. This part of the journey was remarkably quiet.

At the junction of the Falls and Grosvenor roads it was certainly not quiet. A double-decker bus was on fire and a full-scale riot was taking place. A soldier ran towards the car and shouted to us 'get to hell out of here'. In the car we were all in complete panic but we turned right on to the Falls and I was dropped off at the entrance to Bostock House. My father didn't hang about and went on up the Falls. I soon discovered that the gate at Bostock, the Children's Hospital and the rest of the entrances on the Falls were locked. I think I stood for a couple of minutes absolutely terrified but realised I had to carry on walking through the riot to try to get into the hospital from the Grosvenor Road entrance.

I remember so much noise; bricks and petrol bombs were been thrown and paving stones were being pulled up. I don't know if I imagined it but I was sure I had heard shots being fired. I tried my best to look inconspicuous – difficult to do when you are carrying a bright-yellow weekend case – and I felt as if everyone could hear my heart beating. I don't know how I managed to walk as my legs were like jelly but I made it to an unlocked entrance.

Once into the hospital grounds, I felt relieved and reasonably safe, and made my way quickly to Musson House. It was only when I reached there that I started to worry about what had happened to my family and how they got home. I was continually phoning and had to wait a long time before there was an answer. My father told me they had been followed by a black taxi until they reached the outskirts of the city, which he found intimidating.

Over the years we have laughed about the incident, imagining the rioters' and security forces' faces on seeing someone with a bright-yellow case wandering down the road looking as if it was the most normal thing in the world.**

Curfew

"I was on night duty and making my way home via the Grosvenor Road. All of a sudden my car was surrounded by about six soldiers.

'Where do you think you're going?' I was asked, to which I replied 'home'. They told me: 'Don't you know there is a curfew on? You could have been shot.' I said that I was on night duty and wasn't aware of the

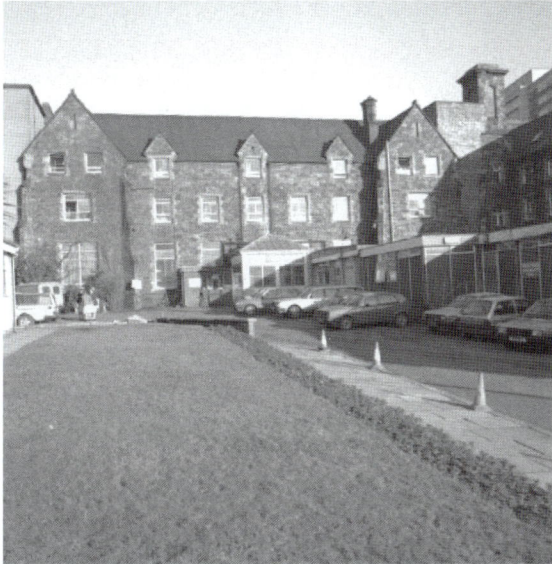

Belfast City Hospital casualty department 1970s

windows of the ambulance were shot in, showering us with glass. Both myself and the doctor lay underneath the two stretchers and the doctor reached his hand up to keep ambu-bagging the patient. My memory is so clear of his hand on the ambu-bag, just bagging away. The ambulance crew kept going and we arrived at the RVH with the patient still alive, and she survived.**"**

A change of mind

"I started my post-registration training in Belfast City Hospital (BCH) in April 1987, having worked previously as a learning disability nurse, and I then accepted a job there.

During the first week in my new post I came off duty and walked to Oxford Street Bus Station to get the bus home. On the way, as the bus headed along the Antrim Road, just beyond Carlisle Circus, it was petrol bombed and hijacked. This was the first time I had ever faced the Troubles so up close and personal.

No one was hurt, but the event made me reflect on my decision to leave my job at the learning disability hospital just five minutes from my home in the country. Back home I would not be required to face the sort of perils I had just encountered. And so I made my life-changing decision to leave general nursing and return to learning disability. I went back to my previous employer and was happily reinstated. I have never had a moment's regret, but I have never admitted the real reason for staying in this branch of nursing.**"**

curfew and that there would be more night nurses leaving the Royal via Grosvenor Road. The soldier in charge asked me if I would mind using the Broadway Exit. I didn't think I had an option. I thanked him for not shooting me and left by Broadway.**"**

Caught in the crossfire

"I was a third-year student nurse in the Belfast City Hospital (BCH) in 1977. I was accompanying a patient who was being transferred from BCH A&E department to the Royal Victoria Hospital intensive care department.

A Malaysian doctor was also in attendance. The patient had been intubated and ambu-bagged using the black rubber type of bag. The ambulance was an old type with small windows. We were almost at the RVH when we were caught in crossfire and the side

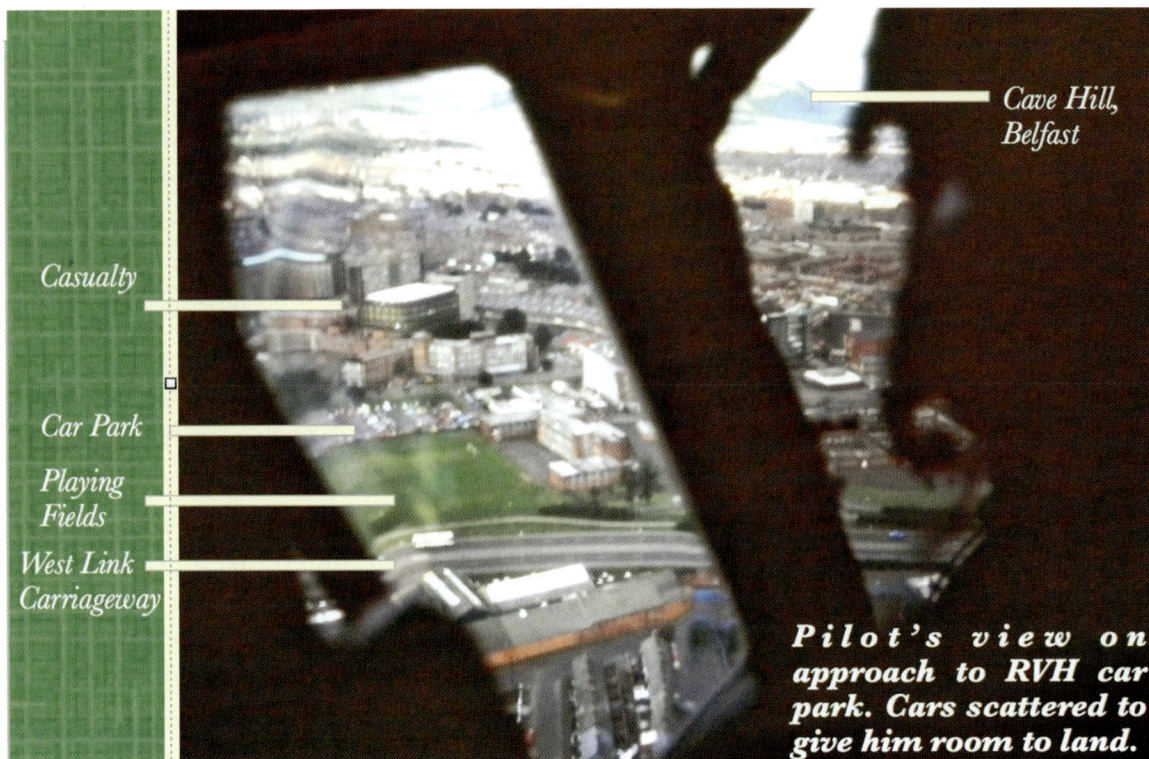

Cave Hill, Belfast

Casualty

Car Park

Playing Fields

West Link Carriageway

Pilot's view on approach to RVH car park. Cars scattered to give him room to land.

Helicopter approach to Royal Victoria Hospital

Using the Ordnance Survey map

❝I started my year's midwifery training in the Royal Maternity Hospital in 1979. As part of the course, I had to undertake a placement with a community midwife in West Belfast working mainly from Ballyowen and Ballymurphy health centres. At that time I was living in nursing accommodation in the hospital complex, so the midwife to whom I was assigned agreed each evening where we would meet up the following morning.

Belfast at this time was experiencing civil unrest and some of the street names had been blanked out or replaced using the Irish language. As I was unfamiliar with the area, I had to buy an Ordnance Survey map to find my way around. By knowing the names and location of the main roads in the area such as Falls, Grosvenor, Springfield and Andersonstown, I was then able to use the map to locate the addresses of the mothers and babies on my caseload list.❞

A flight to remember

❝The late 1970s were a very busy time for anyone working in Altnagelvin Hospital's casualty unit. I was a staff nurse on one late evening shift, during which we had several gunshot wounds, as well as the 'normal' casualties.

A civilian was brought in with a severe gunshot wound to his upper leg and, after assessment both by our surgeons and the Royal Victoria Hospital in Belfast via a phone link, it was decided that the patient should be transferred immediately to the Royal. As time was of the essence, a mode of transport other than ambulance was thought necessary.

One of the casualty officers on duty had good contacts with the British army and, very shortly, we heard the sound of a helicopter landing on the front lawn of the hospital. Initially, we thought we were getting a Wessex, and I was told to prepare to accompany the patient, as I had been on a helicopter flight a few weeks earlier. When I took the patient to the front of the hospital, my heart sank, as I saw that we were to travel in a small four-person craft. How was I going to manage my patient in such cramped conditions, especially as he could be sick after the pethidine injection he had just received? I was glad that I had a vomit bowl with me.

We were hurriedly strapped into the small helicopter, with my very weak patient's head resting on my knees. As the co-pilot was adjusting my throat microphone and headphones, he removed the vomit bowl, telling me to use their sick bags instead. We lifted off into a very dark and wet night and my patient immediately vomited, filling the sick bag. Unfortunately, there was a hole in the bottom of the bag and the contents spilled out, onto my dress and down my legs to my feet. I let out an exclamation and was immediately instructed by the crew not to talk, as it would interfere with their communications. I was so concerned for the welfare of my patient that I tried my best

not to talk again. Unfortunately, childhood memories of my fear of heights, and the ignominy of having to be removed from a 'chair-o-plane' at a fairground, came flooding back. I began to pray quietly but the pilot picked this up and I was again instructed to stay quiet.

When I was a child, my mother had made us hide under the stairs whenever there was thunder and lightning. Ever since, I had a dread of it. I sat there in the dark, afraid even to whisper a prayer, as we flew into a thunderstorm and I wondered how I would cope.

At that point, my patient fell into a drugged sleep and all my time was taken up with monitoring his airway. I kept my hand on his chest, feeling his heart beating, and the movements of his chest, all the time worrying what I would do if he deteriorated.

I soon realised that the crew were newcomers to Derry and unsure of where they were going. They produced a large map and proceeded to spread it over the co-pilot's knees, as they searched for landmarks in the dark, trying to fly along the coast past Coleraine. My confidence in them was dropping by the minute, with their use of the map, and the thunderstorm still booming and flashing around us. Suddenly, we were plunged into pitch darkness and the pilot screamed: 'Jesus Christ, we've hit the mountain!'

There was a moment of silence, followed by the quiet tones of the co-pilot trying to reassure him that what we had actually hit was thick fog. Hearing this, I started audibly praying again, grateful that my patient was unaware of what was going on. However, the pilot shouted at me to shut up and be quiet. Tears flowed down my face as the emotions I had kept in check flooded through me. Seconds earlier, I had thought I was going to die.

Conditions in the air were now so bad that the pilot decided to land the helicopter at Aldergrove army base. We headed there but, just as we were about to land, he changed his mind and took off again. Staying as close to the ground as possible, we headed for Belfast.

City lights

I began to feel some relief as the lights of Belfast started to appear, and hoped that, at last, I would soon be safely on the ground. The crew, however, had other ideas. The map reappeared as they tried to find the Royal Victoria Hospital. Eventually, they located the Falls Road and flew up and down it several times, trying to find the hospital in the darkness. It was at this point that I remembered a news item from a few weeks earlier, about a British army helicopter being shot whilst circling the Falls Road. How much more could I take? How crazy was it to find myself in this position, when I had two young children at home?

Eventually, the crew found a green area, probably a football pitch, and landed. They had already requested that an ambulance meet us, and what a wonderful sight it was! As my patient was being transferred to the ambulance, the helicopter crew approached, telling me to get on board again, as they had received orders to take me back to Derry.

I almost screamed at them, but, instead, quietly said that I would rather walk home than get into the helicopter with them. I jumped into the ambulance and went with my patient to the hospital.

Several hours later, Altnagelvin Hospital sent one of its transport vehicles to the Royal to bring me home. It was well past midnight and my shift was long over when I arrived back at casualty. The first thing to greet me was the body of a very young British soldier, who had been shot somewhere in Derry that night.

I wept for him. He could have been anyone's son, and my traumatic flight was put into perspective. As for the crew of the helicopter, they were also very young, and probably more scared than I was on that flight. But they had helped to save the life of a civilian victim of the Troubles in Derry. **"**

Lighter moments

❝I remember a colleague called Attracta was erroneously named by her Protestant clients unfamiliar with the name as 'Mrs Tractor' or 'Atrixo'. The hilarity this generated amongst community colleagues allowed for open acceptance of religious and cultural differences.❞

Health Visitor

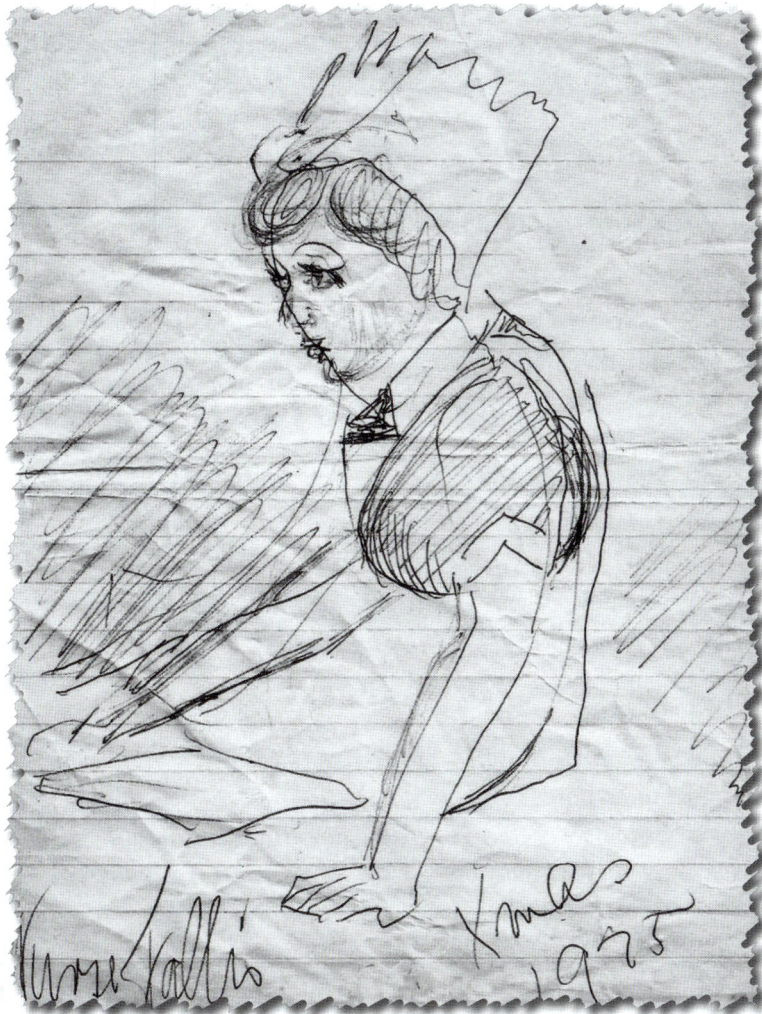

Paramilitary patient's drawing of nurse, 1975

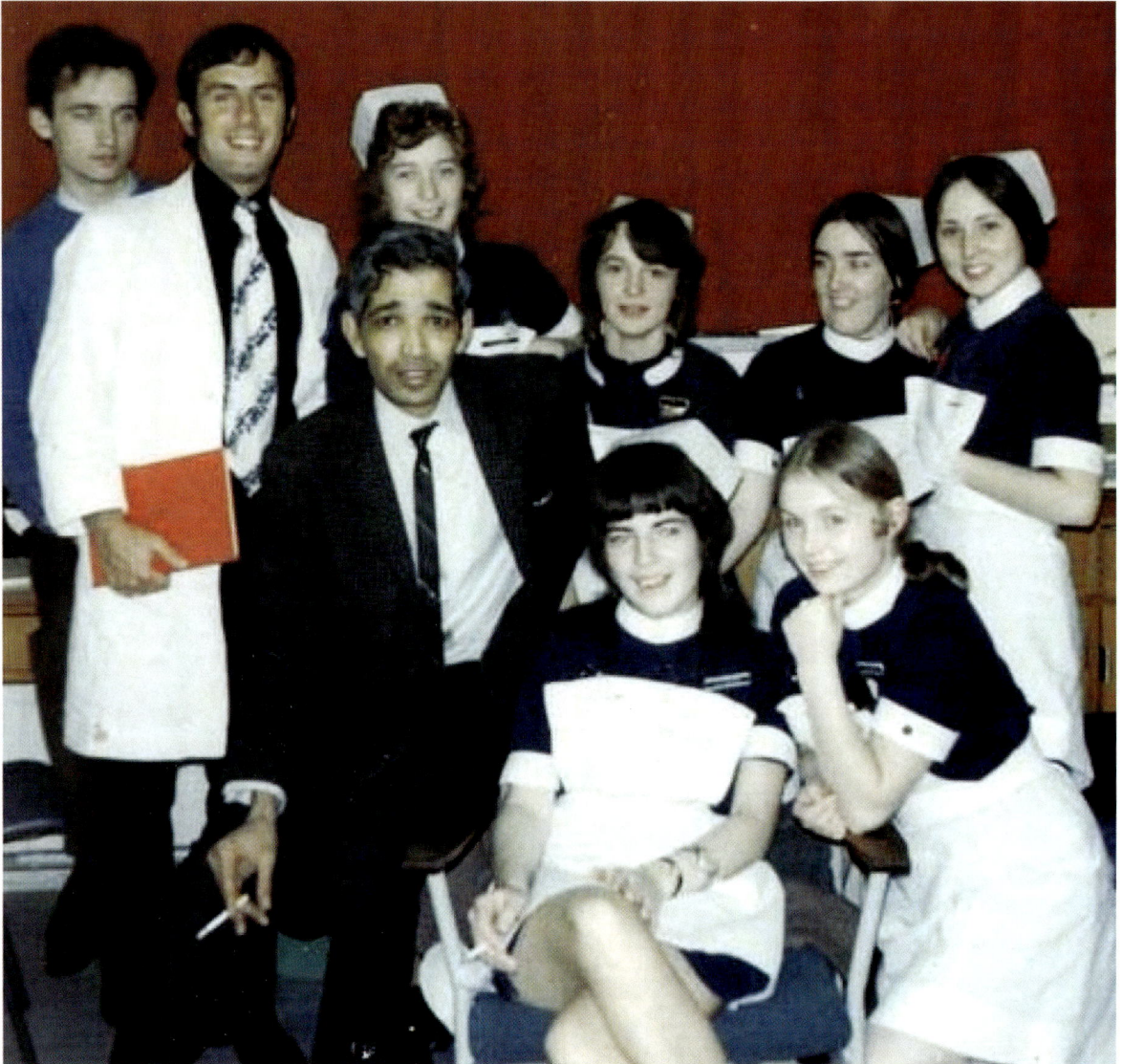

Altnagelvin night duty tea break

In gathering stories, nurses were invited to recount any amusing memories. Many felt that these accounts were too "black" and inappropriate to record, but such is the unique Northern Irish sense of humour, it was often the only way to cope with many bleak situations. Humour was a means of escaping from the reality of a stressful day of trying to cope with the on-going workload in the aftermath of any disturbance which resulted in severe injuries.

The camaraderie generated by finding something to provoke laughter with colleagues was a means of relieving stress, and with student nurses in particular, a way to keep sane when dealing with the old-style authoritarian ward sisters.

The ticking bag

"One of many incidents that stands out in my mind during the Troubles happened in Altnagelvin Hospital on a sunny evening in the summer of 1973, when I was working as a junior staff nurse in casualty.

It was, as usual, a very busy evening and we were dealing with several casualties, when there was a loud knock at the door of the examination/treatment room. Sister opened it to find a young man who seemed distraught. 'I'm sorry to trouble you, but there's a bag in the waiting room and it's ticking.' I immediately went to clear the waiting area as sister phoned to bleep the nursing officer in charge that evening.

After a tense few minutes, the call was returned and sister started to explain our situation. To our shock the nursing officer told sister to take the ticking brown bag out of the waiting area and to leave it outside in case it was a bomb! 'What?' says sister, 'you want me to lift the ticking bag and take it outside?' 'Yes,' she was told, 'Do it now and I will ring the bomb squad.'

We both gasped but, as happened in those days, we did as we were told.

Sister lifted the bag, I cleared the way and we walked out of the department. We didn't know where to put it, so we kept walking as far from the hospital as possible over to a nearby grassy area. Sister put the bag gently on the grass and we raced back towards the casualty entrance where I almost ran into a police car. I knocked on the window and sister said: 'Are you here about the ticking bag?' 'No, we're here about a road traffic accident, to speak to someone who was knocked down,' replied the policeman. We told him that the man had already been discharged. Then, with a smile on his face, he said: 'Let me hear about this ticking bag.' 'No,' I said. 'You're not in the bomb squad.' With that their radio started relaying a message and the second policeman said: 'We are now!'

The first officer then asked: 'Where is this bag?' To which sister replied: 'It's over there in the middle of that grassy area.' He seemed surprised. 'Who took it out there?' 'Me,' said sister, 'following instructions from my Nursing Officer.' To which the officer replied: 'She obviously doesn't think much of you.'

They both left to check the bag, all the while talking on their radios, as we stood our ground at the casualty entrance. A short time later they gave the 'all clear' and came back to us laughing. The first policeman said: 'I have been bombarded with many things in my time, including a nail bomb, but I've never been attacked with a pound of mince and an alarm clock before.'

We guessed that the wee man who had been knocked down went without his supper that night!**"**

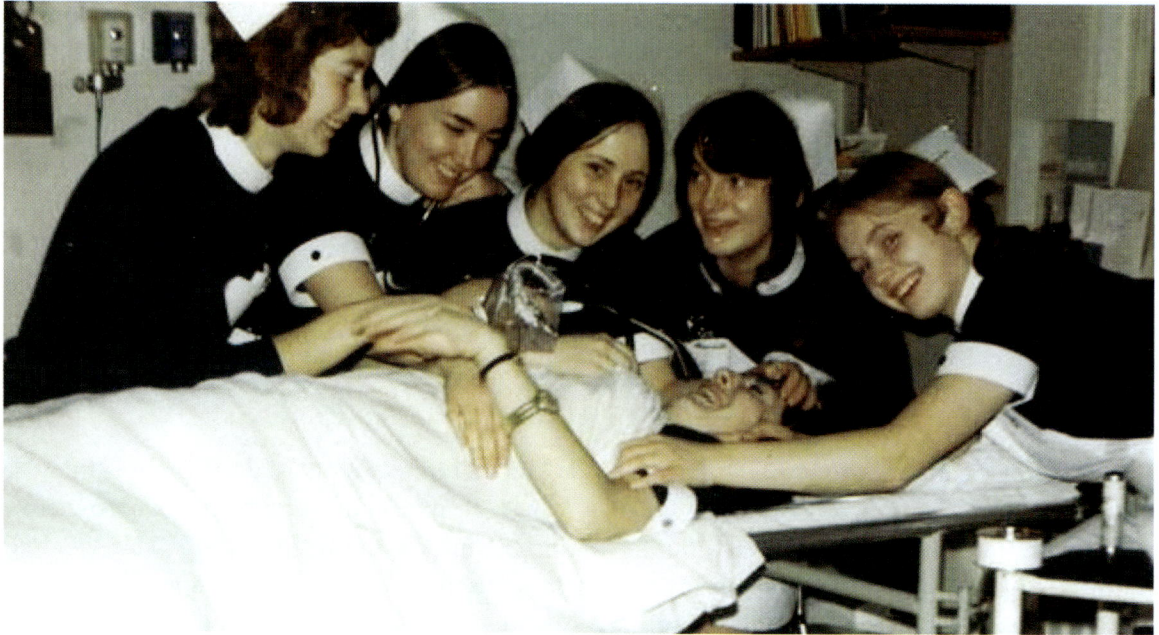

Altnagelvin PTS having fun

Match of the day

"One learns quickly that managing a busy unit takes ingenuity, and sometimes that means breaking the rules.

On my 84-bed unit, critically injured and ill patients in some areas, those who had been 'kneecapped' sometimes for the second, third and, for one poor man, the fourth time, in another.

Elsewhere elderly patients, confused because of their fractures and strange surroundings, police guarding patients, army guarding police and, in the bottom bays, those admitted with sports injuries. Not ill, not even unwell at times, just fractured limbs held in Thomas splints suspended from gantries. Lights-out at 9.30pm/10pm did nothing to ease the sheer boredom of these young men.

In those days Match of the Day, or some other TV programme focusing on sports, was normally scheduled on a Saturday night for about one hour. Unfortunately it was on after lights-out and the Night Matrons normally did their first round about that time as well. The first few hours on night duty are usually the busiest and having one or two bays of bored young men didn't help. Direct action was required.

Following negotiation it transpired that missing Match of the Day was unbearable to this group of patients. Folks from Northern Ireland may be bombing and killing each other wholesale, but when it came to sport, the Union Jack and the Tricolour paled into insignificance compared to Man U beating Liverpool.

The only means of reaching the unit was by stairs or lift. Being near the top of the building meant that everyone, including the Night Matrons, used the lift to access our unit. The deal was made, lights went out, silence reigned, more or less, except when a 'great goal' was scored, cups of tea were provided and quiet, content patients were glued to the small television screen.

The phone rang with a message asking if something was wrong with the lift. 'Sorry Matron, if you hold on I'll just check.' Down the ward, double-time walking, into the bay, TV off, out to the lift, remove the bit of cardboard which was preventing it from leaving the floor, then straight back to the phone. 'No Matron, the lift seems fine.' Ding! The lift arrives; Matron steps out and begins her round. Into the Match of the Day bays, all lights out, all patients sleeping, TV off.

'All very quiet tonight, nurse?' 'Indeed Matron, all quiet.'**"**

The band played on

"During the height of the Troubles in the 1970s, I switched on the television one Sunday morning over breakfast, interested in a news update for the West Belfast area where I worked as a health visitor.

At that moment the announcer was relating that, while there had been serious overnight disturbances, all was now quiet. The cameraman swept up and down the street to prove it. Just at that moment a Salvation Army band flickered into sight marching straight down the middle of the road towards the city centre. Ironically the tune being played was – yes, you've guessed it – 'Onward Christian Soldiers, marching as to war'...**"**

A 'body' in the boot

"Driving along the motorway late one night on the way home to Belfast, I was pulled over to an army checkpoint and asked to show ID and get out of the car.

The young soldier very politely asked me to open my boot and wanted to know where I was coming from. He called some of the squad over.

That is when I began to panic. It was 1971 and I was a student health visitor doing a fieldwork placement in Richhill, County Armagh. My Mini was full of health education paraphernalia such as projectors, boxes of leaflets, charts and anatomical models for antenatal and contraception classes.

Most worrying of all I had a mannequin, used for cardiac/pulmonary resuscitation, squashed in the boot, and I mean squashed. As they approached the boot, guns at the ready, I started to explain that there was this 'thing' in my boot. I was stuck, couldn't think of the word for 'dummy' or 'mannequin', and to my horror blurted out 'there's a… there's a… body in the boot.'

I have never seen men move so fast, their guns pointing at the car. It was eerie and terrifying in the dark with wavering lights and shadows and it was getting cold.

'Open the boot slowly,' he commanded. I was fiddling with the key trying to control my nerves. After what seemed an age the boot popped open and out sprung Resusie Annie into my arms.

'Lay that on the ground and stand back,' he barked. The soldiers gave Annie a good going over and handed her back to me as they took my car apart. One guard stood over me as if I was going to run away.

It was then that the hysteria set in as I stood there hugging Annie for dear life. I watched the soldiers take everything out, including models of female pelvises, various types of contraception and anatomical charts not normally seen on a motorway. I stood there gulping back laughter, shaking and dying to find a toilet.

This scene went on for what seemed an age but probably wasn't that long. Eventually I was allowed to get back into the car. I put Annie beside me as there was no room anywhere else. I felt that after what she had been through she deserved the front seat. The soldier waving me off gave a big smile and a wink. I bet they don't have many car searches like that. **"**

Mind the make-up

"I was a Staff Nurse in A&E at Belfast City Hospital in 1985/86. I was on duty when Lisburn Road Police Station was blown up. Thankfully there were no serious injuries brought to the unit. But in the morning as I walked home up the Lisburn Road with a colleague, she gasped as she saw part of the roof of the house she lived in was gone, exposing her room. Her first concern was for her expensive make-up that she kept by the window.

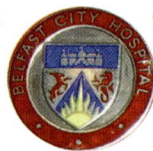

I also worked in A&E with a staff nurse who, when we had any major trauma call alert, would immediately get her compact out with its attached mirror and renew her lipstick. Everyone else would be ensuring that the trauma resuscitation area was ready for the imminent arrivals. She would look up and say, 'You never know'. This became her catchphrase as she was always on the alert for the influx of talent in the form of paramedic crews, the RUC and various other potential husbands. 'You never know' became a mantra of eternal optimism.

I also remember…

Jimmy the Drunk
During my time at the hospital's A&E, there was a 'gentleman of the streets' who was a regular attendee, even in the middle of major disasters. I suspect it was because he liked a bit of company and a warm environment. Let's call him Jimmy. He was also fond of a drink or two. One evening he was making a nuisance of himself in the waiting area. He was harmless but bothering people who were not well, some with children. I went out to the waiting room to remonstrate with him saying: 'Come on Jimmy, you have to stop bothering these people. Sit yourself down and we'll call you in soon.'

But he wasn't playing ball. He continued to invade people's personal space and try to start unwanted conversations, which was not pleasant as he had halitosis and smelt of drink. I said: 'Jimmy if you don't sit down and do as you're told, I'll have to call the RUC again. You don't want that do you?'

He drew himself up to his full height, top hat included, which he always wore, and said very loudly and politely: 'Well, f--- you and f--- the RUC too.' The whole waiting room burst out laughing while I retreated, beetroot faced."

"I'm not gittin' stitched!"

"It wasn't all doom and gloom, and we had many laughs. I remember one time around the July parade season a patient, decked out in his band uniform and pleasantly drunk was brought to A&E after being struck on the head by a police baton.

He had a huge laceration to his head, and his scalp could be lifted to reveal a large area of his skull. He was willing to have his head X-rayed but refused stitches. Me and a colleague, both from different religious backgrounds, tried to persuade him to accept the treatment and explained why it was essential that he had the wound closed. He tried hard to think up good reasons why he wouldn't comply.

His best excuse was: 'No I'm not gittin stitched. I'd become a Catholic first!'

Both of us looked at each other and burst out laughing. We kept a close eye on him and let him have a sleep for a while and did central nervous system observations. Later he fortunately consented to treatment."

A patient's humour

A nurse from the Royal intensive care unit recalls…

"A policeman had received a severe gunshot wound to his head, removing a large portion of his skull. The wound was debrided and a titanium graft and skin graft performed. He made an unexpected recovery, and though left paraplegic, seemed to be mentally unimpaired.

Following his transfer from intensive care, one of the consultants went to see him in the ward where his wife was visiting. The consultant asked him what hospital he was in and he replied that it was the Mater. His wife said: 'Come on, you know you are not in the Mater.' His response was: 'Well, if the doctor doesn't know what hospital he's in, I'm not going to tell him!'"

The red bus

A midwife remembers:

"A red bus was spotted in the wee small hours adjacent to the wing of the Royal Maternity Hospital, opposite the tennis courts. All the lights of the bus were ablaze with the door wide open.

By this stage the natural suspicion had to be that there was a bomb on board. Security was informed and immediate preparation for the evacuation of three floors commenced. It was a great relief when security phoned to say that there was a simple explanation. A driver had taken his sick colleague to A&E. Little did he know the anxiety he caused. But we were able to laugh about this later. **"**

"Nurse, tell them to stop rioting!"

A community nurse recalls…

"Dealing with the unexpected was all too common. One of my duties along with a colleague from the housing estates on the opposite side of the Springfield Road was running a joint child health clinic. This was a popular rendezvous for mothers, babies and toddlers on Monday afternoons.

On one occasion a very nasty incident erupted a few hundred yards away on waste ground behind the clinic. This may have been sparked off by a security forces search of some nearby houses. When I went out to investigate the commotion, the army – at least eight to ten soldiers in full riot gear – was charging a large angry mob of residents, mostly men and youths who were reciprocating with pavement stones, bricks, bottles and so on.

These missiles were coming over the clinic roof and landing on the parked, but fortunately empty, prams outside. Since my colleague and I feared that road closures were imminent, not to mention the risk of tear gas to disperse the mob, we decided to evacuate the clinic as quickly and safely as possible.

Ironically while I was outside helping the mothers to get packed up and away, one

mum said: 'Nurse why don't you two go and tell them to stop rioting until we get out of here?'

Naturally we did not act on this, only too well aware that our nursing skills did not rise to quelling angry mobs when emotions were running high. **"**

Let sleeping soldiers lie

"I was a charge nurse in the operating theatres in Craigavon Hospital. It was the early 1970s and the hospital had been open for about a year. The operating theatre consisted of the operating rooms and a recovery ward where patients spent some time after their surgery to wake up from their anaesthetic and then return to their ward. The intensive care unit (ICU) was just across from the theatre and had only six beds in those days.

Sometimes the recovery ward was used for longer term nursing of patients who needed intensive care and monitoring when there were insufficient beds in the ICU. On other occasions it was used to nurse soldiers or policemen who would normally have gone to a ward, but in the recovery ward it was a little easier to provide security for them.

An injured soldier who had been in surgery was being nursed in the recovery ward with one of his colleagues on guard duty just outside the clinical area. The guard was in full combat uniform and had a rifle. I was on night duty – in those days the Theatre Sisters and Charges Nurses all took turns at doing night duty.

We had provided a chair for the soldier on guard duty so he could sit inside the theatre department but outside the recovery room. The operating theatre staff were having a tea break at about three or four o'clock in the morning and I made tea and toast for the soldier on guard. I took it out to him but found him asleep in his chair with the rifle across his knees.

I went up and spoke to him, touching his shoulder. He jumped out of his seat clearly very alarmed at being woken up, and the rifle was pressed very close to my head. Fortunately he did not pull the trigger and I was very relieved when he woke up fully and realised where he was and that I posed him no threat. He was very apologetic and remained awake for the rest of his duty.

I resolved never again to approach a sleeping soldier!**"**

Buns and biscuits on the motorway

A nurse lecturer remembers…

"Commuting to and from work during the Troubles was often a slow and frustrating process. By the mid 1970s I was living in the Castlereagh area but travelling to the then Polytech Jordanstown, where I was a lecturer in health visiting.

Frequently on the homeward journey we ended up parked on the eight-lane motorway while bombs and bomb scares were dealt with in Corporation Street. On one memorable summer evening while we were thus marooned for nearly four hours, I witnessed the following incident.

A gentleman got out of the car next to mine and crossed over to an Ormo Bakery bread van a couple of lanes away. After a hasty conversation, the breadman also left his van, opened the doors and in no time at all was selling cakes, buns and biscuits to a hungry horde of car and truck drivers. Business opportunities can crop up anywhere! It certainly lightened the atmosphere of an otherwise frustrating hold-up.**"**

Last Rites

A casualty nurse's story…

"Despite, or perhaps because of, the strain of that time, there were many funny incidents which helped to keep us all going. Most of these could not be repeated, certainly not in writing, but one or two stand out.

It was standard practice to send for the Roman Catholic (RC) hospital Chaplain in the event of an admission of someone whose injuries were serious, either if he or she was known to be RC or if the denomination was not known. Having long given up watching the local news, I was not always familiar with the appearance of many of our leading political activists.

One day, when dealing with a victim of the violence in the resuscitation room, I said to the senior sister that I was 'just going to ring the priest'. I thought she looked at me rather strangely and she quietly mouthed the patient's name, which meant nothing to me. When she saw my bewilderment she repeated it, but I still couldn't understand what his name had to do with it, and went on down to the office to use the phone. As I lifted the receiver, she arrived, rather breathless, in my wake and told me to put the phone down. Apparently, the man was an extremely well-known Loyalist paramilitary."

A bow to the bishop

"In casualty we were often visited by famous people and on one occasion were told that the then Archbishop of Canterbury, Dr Donald Coggan, was about to pay us a call.

On the morning of the event, one of the doctors and myself were discussing arrangements with the Church of Ireland Chaplain, when a certain non-conformist nursing colleague became increasingly irritated by the whole thing and complained that it was ridiculous to make such a fuss of an 'ordinary' man.

This led to some straight-faced leg-pulling in which we informed her that she should really curtsy to the great man on arrival, and not to do so would simply betray her own ignorance. Casualty then became very busy over the next hour or so and we forgot all about the conversation until, being the most senior nurse on duty, she was called to go along with the consultant and welcome our illustrious visitor. Apparently, she made him a very low curtsy indeed. It was only later, when she had seen me merely shake hands with the Archbishop, that she realised it had been a 'wind-up'!"

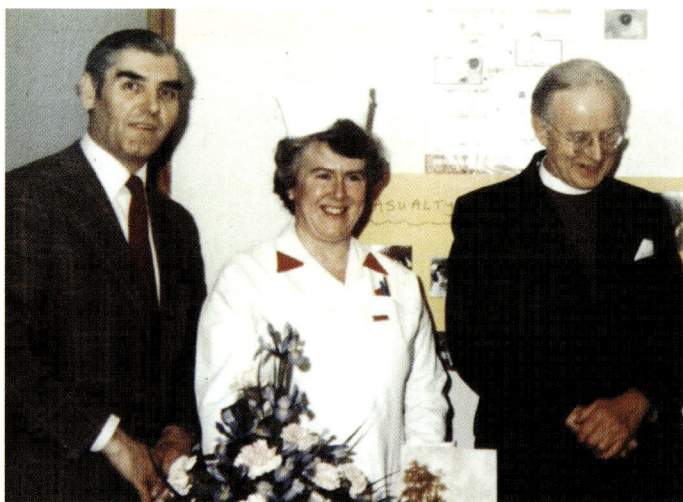

A visit by the Archbishop of Canterbury

"Sammy Sammy!"

A sister at Musgrave Park Hospital remembers:

"A particular incident which I recall with some amusement was a telephone call I received around 9.30pm on the Saturday evening following the bombing incident at Musgrave Park Hospital in 1991.

This call came from the mother of an eight-year-old boy Jack, who had been discharged on the Friday before the bombing.

His mother was anxious to know if everyone was safe and well. She reported that while she was in her kitchen preparing the evening meal her son, who had been watching television, shouted loudly for her attention: 'Mammy, mammy they're all dead in Musgrave Park!' He was anxious in particular about his friend Sammy who had remained as an inpatient. The boys were both the same age and had become friendly, sharing an interest in football. Having reassured his mother that we were all well, she asked if they could come up to visit the next day.

Just after lunchtime on Sunday the family appeared with Jack who was mobilising with his rollator. On reaching the office, he looked down the ward and spied his friend Sammy; he immediately abandoned the rollator and crawled on his knees the short distance to Sammy's bed. He pulled himself up, holding on the siderail of the bed and stared at the other eight year old, full of genuine concern. He said: 'Sammy, Sammy, I thought you was dead!' To which Sammy replied, with some irritation and embarrassment, 'Well I'm nat so I'm nat!' in a flat Belfast accent. The onlookers smiled and some laughed out loud.

This event is memorable and also touching because these two boys were from different cultures and had become friends in a hospital setting when, sadly, in a divided community they would have been unlikely to meet in the normal course of events.**"**

The toilet entourage

An outpatient Sister recalls...

"My clerical assistant and I were delegated the task of arranging the outpatients appointments for the prisoners.

There were usually two prison officers with the prisoner who was handcuffed to both of them – one on each side. There were two policemen guarding the prison officers. Bringing up the rear were two soldiers whose responsibility it was to ensure the safety of the policemen.

More often than not the prisoner would request to use the toilet. Needless to say, the toilets in outpatients were not built for such an entourage, and the clanging of the handcuffs could be heard down the corridor."

Four in the morning

From a staff nurse living in the Towers...

"There was an army lookout post opposite the Towers. One night we were on our way home from a dance in Ballymena but the taxi wouldn't come up Broadway.

So there we were at 4am walking along Broadway cheerfully shouting up at the army. There had been shooting just one hour before. Looking back now I think: how crazy were we...?"

Working alongside weapons

"I remember the night we were going to be blown up. We were all drinking coffee and tea – maybe others were having slurps! – here we were drinking tea and we were going to be blown up!"

Matron, Royal Victoria Hospital

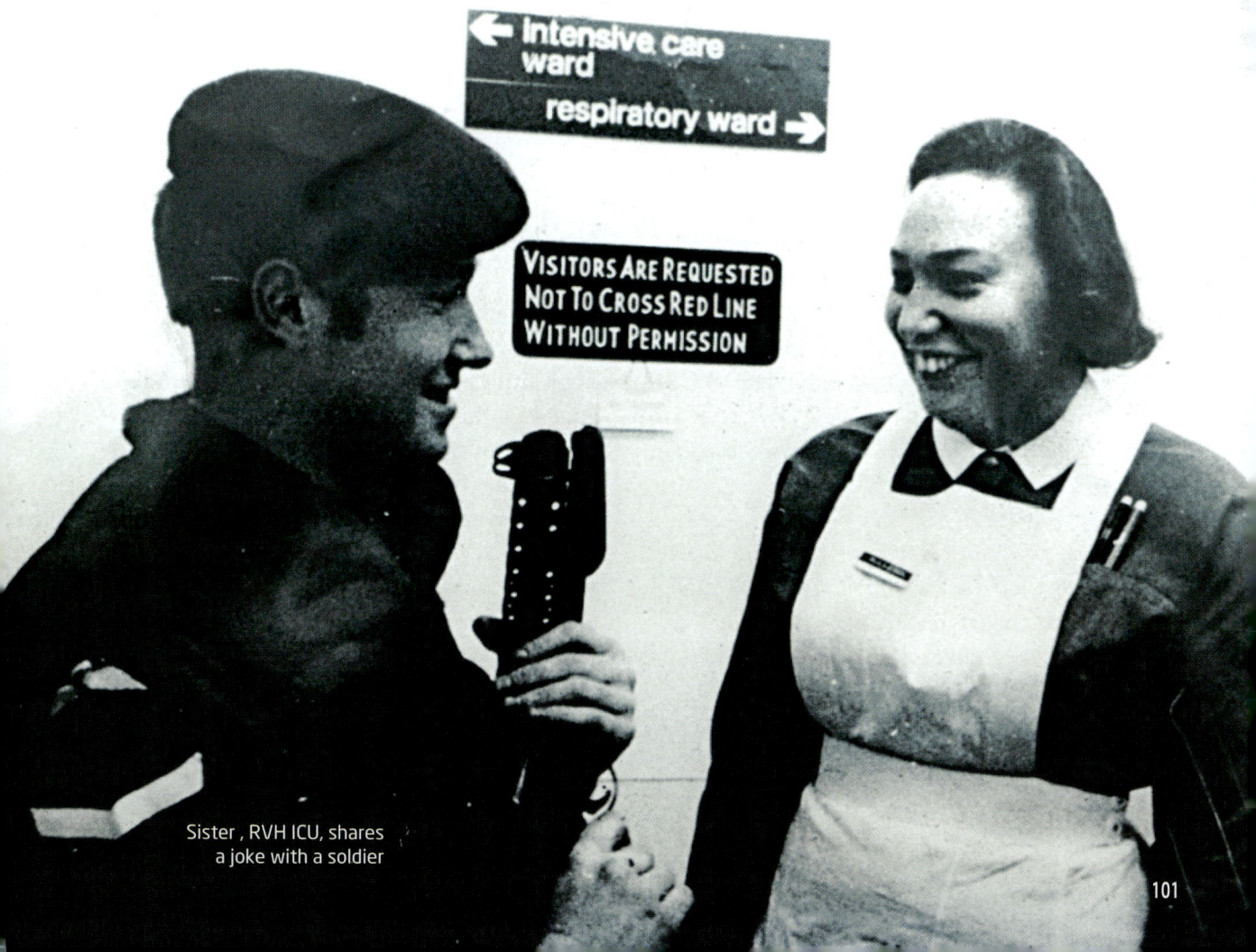

Sister , RVH ICU, shares
a joke with a soldier

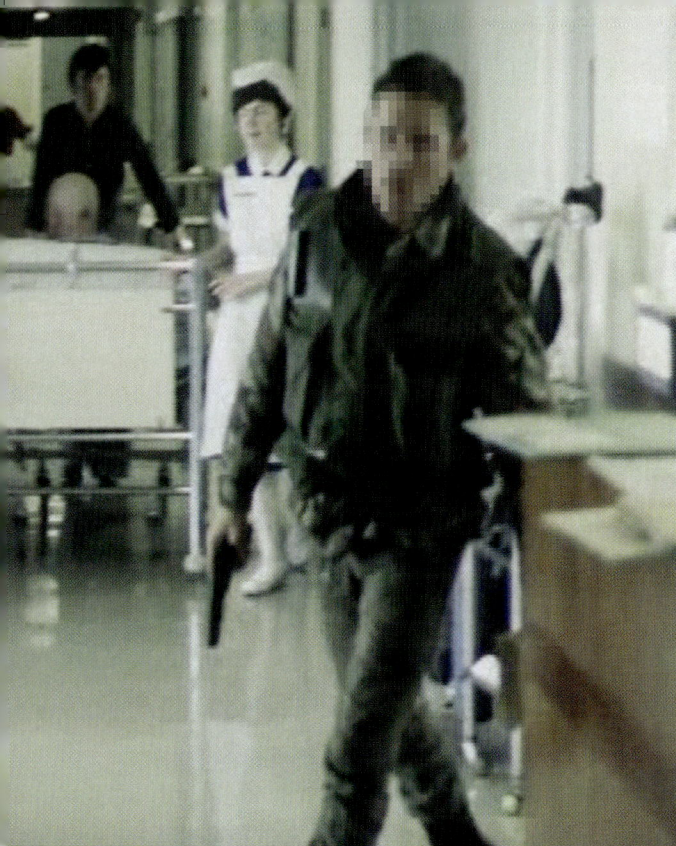
Soldier with gun at nurses' station, RVH

©BBC

"I asked a nurse had she nothing better to do than stand beside a bin. 'The police asked me to guard it,' she said. When I looked in it was full of their weapons and the policemen were having a cuppa!"

Night Sister, Royal Victoria Hospital

"In resuscitation police used to set down guns. We were tripping over guns. Looking back it was unbelievable."

Staff Nurse, Craigavon Area Hospital

Visiting times had their own complexities as relatives of opposing patients could cause mayhem. Another unexpected dilemma for nurses included patients who made a dash for freedom. Escapes were frequently planned by those under guard, much to the horror of the nurses looking after them. Every hospital had an escapee!

Ward corridors became crowded places when patients were guarded by members of the police and army. Patients from the security forces had an armed guard for protection as did those patients suspected of paramilitary activity. It was not uncommon for police, army and paramilitary patients to be beside each other, nor was it uncommon for paramilitaries from "either side" to be in a ward next to each other. At times, some staff were targeted as well.

Injured police or army personnel had to have their weapons safely removed by a weapons expert to prevent accidental discharge of bullets when admitted to casualty. Nurses remembered becoming accustomed to passing security personnel with rifles in wards, canteens and passageways. Such scenes heightened anxiety levels for all concerned, including relatives.

Hostile relations

❝I remember while working in the neurosurgery ward someone with severe head injuries was admitted. He was under guard by the army with two soldiers at the door of the side room at all times. The family found this difficult and hostile feelings were evident.

I became involved inadvertently. I and another student were tending to this patient's pressure areas. He was unconscious but at times during interventions would become unsettled and aggressive. On one occasion we had difficulty carrying out our task. When we had turned him on his side he became difficult to manage and almost fell out of bed. We were in the room with the door closed and neither of us could let go of him to reach for the nurse call buzzer, so we shouted as loud as we could for help.

I suppose the soldiers must have heard the panic in our voices and they came into the room and helped us move the patient away from the edge of the bed and replace the cot sides.

Just at that moment some family members appeared and we were subjected to verbal abuse. This carried on for some time and when we were walking off duty some time later we met some of the family at the exit from the hospital. We were verbally abused and were pushed and shoved by them. They pulled at our capes trying to read our name badges. We pushed our way through and hurried to the safety of the nurses' home.

We were both terrified after this incident and although I have always done so, I have never felt comfortable wearing a name badge since. **"**

Carry on as usual

"I was working on night duty in the neurosurgery ward in the Royal Victoria Hospital; there were actually two wards although there was only one nursing station where the two wards met. There had been an incident in a police station earlier resulting in a man sustaining a severe head injury. He had been admitted to the ward where he was nursed in a side room under guard by the army at all times.

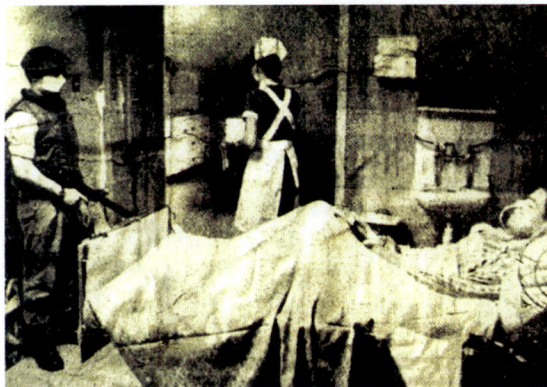
Nurse and soldier with gun at hospital bed

On this particular night when I went on duty, part of the handover was to be given by an army officer and before he spoke we were not sure why. We were told there had been an incident at the home of the consultant treating the patient and it was felt by the security forces that the IRA may try to take him from the ward that night.

It felt like the entire army was in the ward, but strangely this was not reassuring. We were told that there were extra security forces in the hospital and it was highly unlikely that any intruder would actually reach the ward. Nevertheless we were given instructions as to what we should do if this situation arose. We had to move all the patients from the side of the ward where this man was being nursed. I think we gave water leaking through the ceiling as the reason. It wasn't nice having to lie to our patients but we had been told they must not find out the real reason. All the staff were feeling vulnerable and afraid, but we had to carry on as usual.

On night duty I worked in the nursery located in this ward, which was closer to

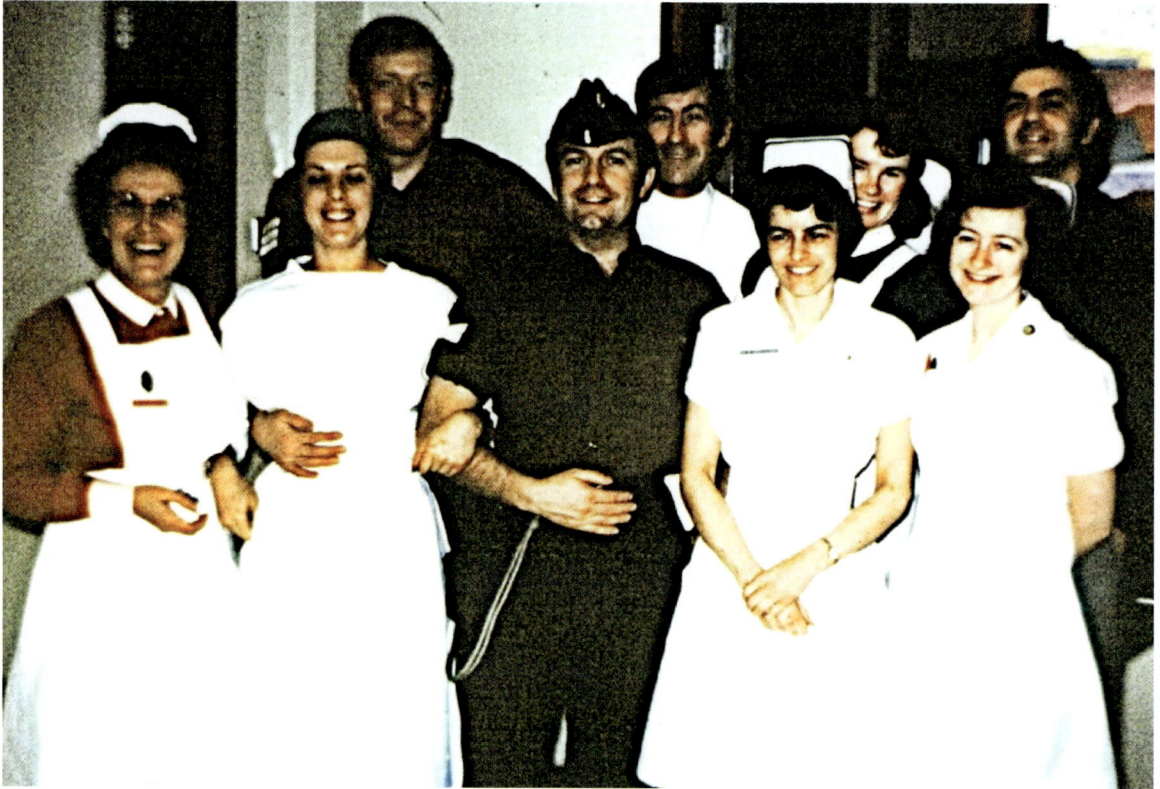

Fracture clinic 1970s

the lift than the rest of the ward. I was given extra instructions as I would have been the first member of staff to encounter any unwelcome visitors. This alarmed me even more. There were four babies in the nursery that night, although none was critically ill. I had to keep the light to a minimum and be as quiet as possible. Unfortunately the babies were quite noisy in the early part of the night.

I moved the cots so they were all at the back of the ward and I planned to place myself between them and the door to the ward, which I had to keep ajar. I worked quickly and all the babies settled to sleep. With this done my whole focus was on what might happen; every ten minutes felt like an hour.

I continually checked the babies hoping to be right beside them when they woke and before they would cry and managed this reasonably well.

A couple of times during the night the lift would beep as it reached our floor making my heart miss a beat or two and I slid down my chair a bit in the hope I wouldn't be spotted. The night wore on slowly and I remember I kept looking out the window to see if it would soon be morning,

I was so relieved when I saw the sun rising a little as I felt that the threat was over. The rest of the morning passed as usual and we went off duty exhausted but very relieved. **"**

A wrong turn of phrase

"A male civilian who had been shot, died in my ward. Two male relatives came to ask about what they had to do.

I explained that as it was a coroner's case, the funeral could not be arranged without his or her agreement. When they enquired further, I said that any case of accidental death had to be reported to the coroner. They immediately became aggressive, shouting that it was not an accident, that he had been shot. I immediately apologised saying that I had used the wrong word, and that I should have said 'any death not from natural causes'. They left, still angry.

Later that day, three very threatening men came to the ward and accused me of trying to pass the death off as an accident. I apologised again for my misuse of the word accident, and assured them that all patients were treated equally and we did not always know the circumstances of their injuries. They appeared mollified and left. It was of great concern to me that they had the impression that I would be able to influence the outcome of such a case. It certainly taught me to choose my words carefully.**"**

A terrified man

"I was on placement in accident & emergency at Lagan Valley Hospital, Lisburn. If a prisoner needed surgery they were treated in the side surgical wards under guard. It was early evening and quiet in the department. A member of the security forces in uniform came in with his son.

The boy had fallen off his bicycle and cut his knee. The wound needed stitches and as I was setting up for this the doctor came to the cubicle and told me the IRA were up in the surgical ward to remove one of their members who was a prisoner admitted for treatment. The doctor told me to stay in the cubicle as they might come through the department on their way out.

The boy's father became hysterical. He started shouting that they were going to shoot him when they saw him in uniform. I tried to reassure him that if he kept quiet and stayed in the cubicle he would be alright. He grabbed me and, holding me in front of him as a shield, he dragged me down the corridor. I couldn't get away and one of his arms was across my throat so tightly I couldn't speak. He kept saying that I wasn't to let them shoot him.

The doctor came back and shouted at him to let me go. He wouldn't, and the doctor had to wrestle me away from him. He gave off to the man telling him I was only a young girl and he had no right to hurt me. The doctor pushed us into a room. He warned the man not to touch me again and told me not to open the door to anyone until he came back. I tried to comfort his son. After a while the doctor came to let us out. He said the gang had left the hospital with the prisoner.

It was a very upsetting incident so early in my training. I was thankful that the man and his son were safe. In the surgical ward the armed gang threatened the staff warning them not to contact the police. They left with the prisoner but thankfully no one was hurt.**"**

'Evacuation of troops or patients advisable'

Sept 72.

Provos warn Army to quit RVH grounds ..or else

THE 2nd Battalion of the Provisional IRA last night announced "the right of assault on the Royal Victoria Hospital and its adjacent quarters occupied by the British forces ... any type of attack is now possible. An evacuation of troops or patients is advisable."

In a statement the I.R.A. warned: "In our forthcoming operations we will ensure that none but the enemy suffer. The British have chosen a hospital grounds as a battlefield; any resulting casualties are their responsibility."

The statement said it declared the right of assault because the Falls Road hospital "has now entered the character of a fortress and is no longer definable as a neutralised zone."

The statement continued: "Hitherto, it has been used as a base for raids and attacks on the surrounding Free Areas. More recently its annexes, and especially the new extension, have been employed beyond an intolerable advantage for the British. Our intelligence reports have definitely established that

1—British patrol groups scan the Lower Grosvenor, Upper Cavendish Street area and the high rise of Beechmount from the new extension using high-powered binoculars and on one such occasion a mounted telescope.

2—that the neutralized zone is exploited by the British for hiding, and in a secret room of the hospital reception is the British Intelligence and RUC Special Branch Sub-Headquarters and finally,

3—that hospital security made act in collusion with the soldiers in the arrangement and co-ordination of patrols.

Patiently we have waited and restrained ourselves from reprisals ... in the vainly hoping that the authorities would ...

not used for any purpose which deprive these ... of protection ... with Article ...

'Onus on IRA'

In the event of casualties as a result of battle at the R.V.H. British Army will undoubtedly lay the onus on the IRA believing that were liable ... the IRA there would ... need for their deployment ... the area.

Commenting last night on the IRA statement, a British ...

NEWS LETTER

Telephone 44441

Tuesday, September 12, 1972

CITY FINAL

Price 3p (4p in Eire)

Clear hospital fortress—warning

IRA THREAT TO ATTACK R.V.H.

News Letter reporter

IRA Provisionals last night warned the Army in Ulster to stop using the Royal Victoria ... a fortress—or face increased attacks on it ... atum said: "Any type of attack is now ... evacuation of patients or troops is ... advisable."

The Provo spokesman said the Army ... had chosen the hospital grounds ... battlefield." They had also ...

Gunmen dressed as doctors carry out daring dawn raid

IRA GANG SNATCHES SICK COMRADE FROM RVH WARD 10

By Martin Lindsay, David Neely and John Conway

AN IRA GANG dressed with submachine guns and revolvers forced their way into the Royal Victoria Hospital in Belfast early yesterday morning and snatched away a comrade who was shot by the Army three days ago.

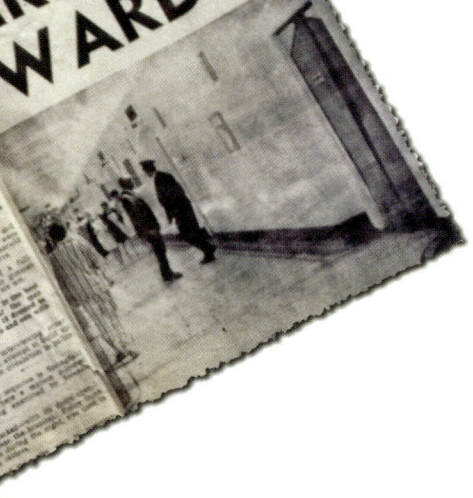

Provos say: We did it

Doubts about security

Daily Mirror

BRITAIN'S BIGGEST DAILY SALE

Tuesday, September 12, 1972   No. 21,334

"We declare the right of assault on the Royal Victoria Hospital .. Evacuation of troops or the patients is advisable" - PROVOS

TERROR THREAT TO A HOSPITAL

By CHRIS BUCKLAND

THE Provisional IRA warned last night that Ulster's biggest hospital, which has 1,200 patients, is now open to any type of attack by them.

Gunmen in the Mater

❝The son of one of our surgeons at the Mater was abducted on his way home from the hospital, tortured and murdered by a Loyalist gang.

Another surgeon was attacked by a Loyalist gang as he left his sons at school. One of the sons was killed and another injured. The doctor suffered a gunshot wound to his arm.

On another occasion three student nurses were targeted as they walked up the street outside the hospital; fortunately they escaped with only one receiving a minor gunshot injury.

Loyalist gunmen walked into an eight-bed ward of patients and sprayed it with gunfire, shooting dead their intended victim, a prominent Republican politician, as well as injuring two other patients.❞

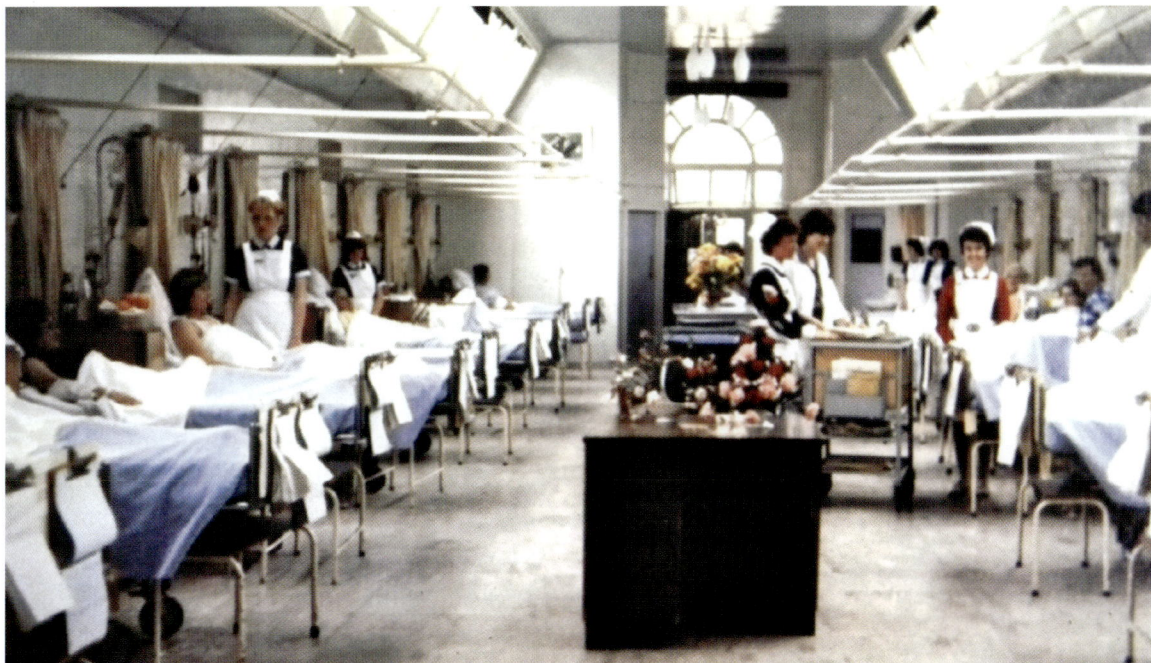

Nightingale ward in the 1970s

Losing a patient

❝By 1973, I had qualified and was working as a staff nurse in a surgical ward. After the morning report, I set about my duties and, following the medicine round, I advised a patient who was first day post-op that he had to have a bath.

For those who are not familiar with the old nightingale wards, the bathroom was located near the entrance to the ward, opposite the nurses' station, and the toilets were at the other end of the ward, in this case beside a balcony. I helped the patient, who was a prisoner, get ready for his bath but before we reached the bathroom, he asked if he could use the toilet. I said 'of course' and we turned to walk towards the toilets. As we approached the toilet door, he ran for the balcony, opened the door and jumped over the rail onto the path underneath. He was last seen running up the Grosvenor Road wearing only his pyjamas and no shoes or slippers.

The interesting thing is that this patient was a prisoner, being guarded by prison officers and police who were standing at the other end of the ward. They saw what had just happened and obviously could do very little. As you can imagine I was left in a state of panic and shock that I had lost a patient.

Later that morning I was interviewed by the police but thankfully I was not considered a serious accomplice to the escape.**"**

Detainee escapes in pyjamas

TROOPS FLOODED the Falls and areas of Belfast this morning to hunt for who escaped from the Royal Victo dressed in his pyjamas.

UVF prisoner flees RVH down drainpipe

A 28-year-old Belfast man serving an eight year jail sentence escaped from a security ward of the Royal Victoria Hospital, last night.

I'm only an old nurse, and what's the good of shooting me?

Miss Gaw writes...

Miss Gaw, RVH

"I was in the corridor after completing the round in one ward when a junior nurse came flying down into the nurses' station saying: 'Sister! Gunman! Gunman!' 'Where,' I asked? 'The side ward,' she said.

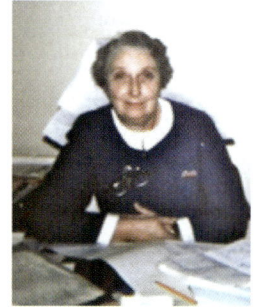

So the senior nurse and I both hurried through the nurses' station, and we saw two people in the side ward. I thought the guard was 'frisking' the person who had come in, but it was vice versa! The nurse in the next ward heard the commotion and called out: 'They've gone that way with the patient.'

As I reached the door the intruder came charging toward me with a gun and shouted: 'Stop or I'll shoot!' Well naturally I stopped. He seemed very nervous, and he was looking all around. A thousand thoughts were passing through my mind: 'I should be inside. I wonder what's happening? How am I to get out of here?' So I gently pushed back one foot, and then the other; he saw me moving slightly, and said: 'I will shoot.'

'Well,' I said, 'I'm only an old nurse, and what's the good of shooting me?' I immediately turned on my heel and went flying back up the ward corridor. I arrived out onto the main corridor, just in time

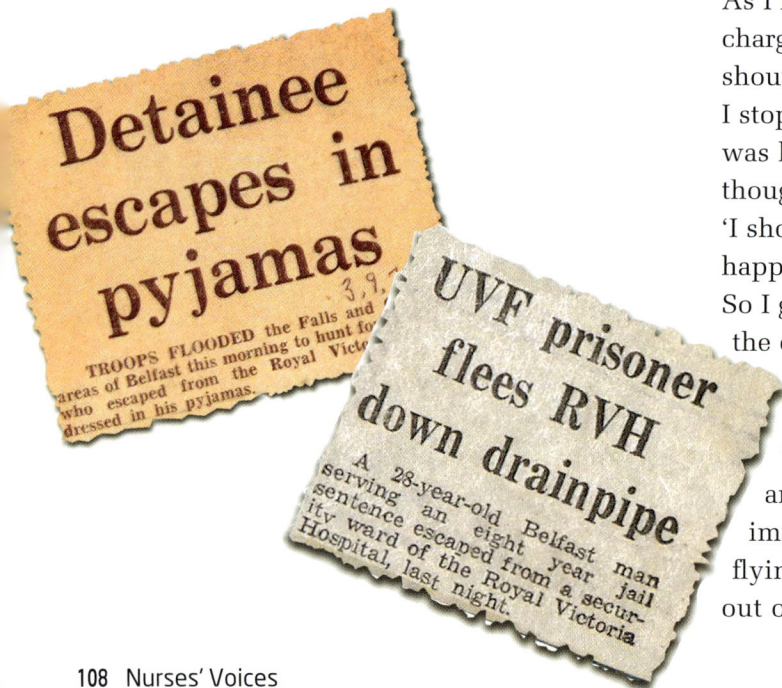

to see the other gunmen walking away dressed in white coats and with guns in their hands. After that the police and security people took over.”

The British army and the wrong Musgrave Hospital, Belfast

“One day a middle-aged man was admitted from the mobile cardiac ambulance following a severe coronary thrombosis. He was a known member of the Official IRA.

Over a period of a week to ten days his condition improved and he was medically ready for transfer to a convalescent bed in the Musgrave and Clarke clinic. This facility had both private and NHS patients and was approximately 200 yards from the cardiology ward and could be easily seen from the far end of the ward.

It was agreed that the transfer would take place early one evening and that the ambulance would be escorted by an armoured personnel carrier for the short door-to-door transfer. An armed soldier arrived to provide the escort out to the ambulance and said: 'We are taking him to the Musgrave Park Hospital.' This hospital is a civilian hospital with a military wing about three miles from the Royal Victoria Hospital. I immediately realised there was confusion over the name of the hospital and the patient was going to be transferred to the wrong place. This would have been very stressful for the man and could have induced another coronary thrombosis.

I explained to this tall, broad, armed soldier – I am 5ft 2in – that a mistake had been made and that I was not prepared to allow the patient to be transferred to the wrong hospital. The soldier shouted, swore and tried to bully me, but I would not agree to the transfer, having telephoned the consultant to explain the reason for my decision.

The other patients were now well aware of what was going on as the office opened directly on to the top end of the ward. When the soldier eventually left, in a very disgruntled manner, I seem to remember a round of applause from the patients. How much of the commotion the patient heard from the cubicle he was in I do not know. I explained to him that he could not be transferred that evening due to the confusion and he remained on the ward until his transfer back to prison.

One of the patients in the side ward was a minister of religion and I understood that he wrote to the hospital mangers about the 'disgraceful way the ward sister had been treated'. I do not recall being contacted by either the managers or the army and I did not mention the difficulties I had had to the patient.

Looking back I feel that I had very mixed emotions at the time. I was cross and frustrated that the soldier would not listen to me when I was in the right and trying to act professionally. I was a bit shaken, though certainly not tearful, as a result of this soldier shouting and trying to bully me. I was also rather pleased that I had done the right thing by my patient and fulfilled my duty of care in challenging circumstances.”

Bank robbery at the RVH

"It started as a routine ward round in January 1973 on the cardiology ward, when I found myself involved in a violent and potentially dangerous situation. I heard gunfire as I went to collect a patella hammer from a trolley at the office end of the ward near the entrance hall to the hospital. I was a Junior Sister on the ward at that time.

The entrance hall had a black and white tiled floor and domed roof. On entering the hospital foyer there was a waiting room to the right and on the left a chaplain's office and a bank office. It emerged that before a doctor and I arrived on the scene, the chaplains had been locked in their office by three armed bank robbers who were holding up the bank staff and the queue of mainly domestic staff who were waiting to be paid.

Unknown to the bank robbers the small British army unit based in the hospital had been alerted to the situation by the chaplains, using the phone in their office. The men were leaving the entrance hall as the army arrived and, as the robbers ran out of the hall towards the street, one of them was shot with an automatic gun and fell to the ground while the other two ran on and escaped. I remember the 30 or so staff screaming in terror when the shooting was occurring, the sounds echoing around the domed roof of the entrance hall.

I went to fetch a transporting trolley kept in the waiting room so, with help, the injured robber was lifted on to the trolley and quickly wheeled into the cardiology ward corridor adjacent to a resuscitation trolley. Basic life support measures were started immediately and he was intubated. Many more staff, including administrators, continued to arrive. The man had five gunshot wounds to his body and I was surprised that there was so little obvious blood loss. He had been gasping when I first saw him but despite strenuous and sustained efforts by the medical and nursing staff, he died about ten minutes after the shooting.

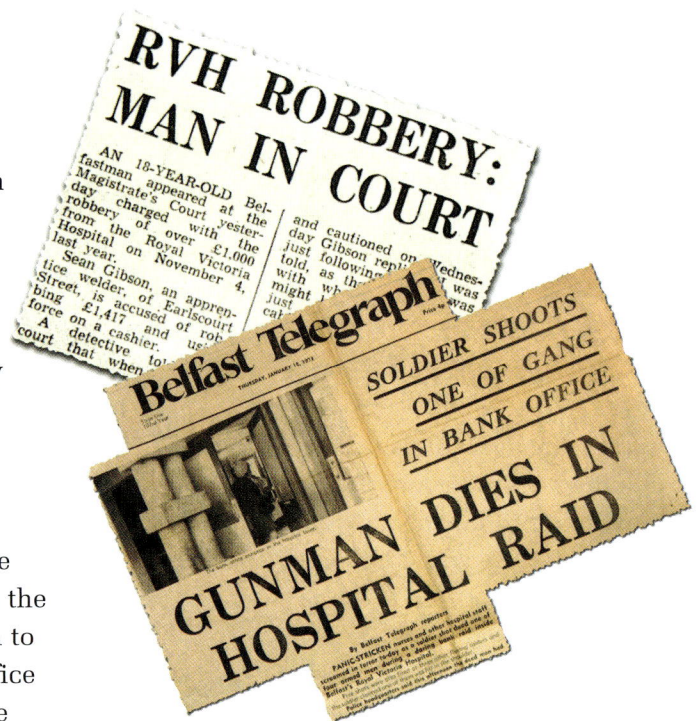

Once the patient was pronounced dead his body was moved into a small clinical room off the ward corridor. I stayed in the room with the body and an armed British soldier. The soldier was there because patients had previously been removed from the hospital by armed paramilitaries. The army private assumed that I knew the man and his name. I was outraged at the implication that everyone in Ulster was close to one of the paramilitary organisations.**"**

The fire at Long Kesh Prison

A Royal Victoria Hospital student nurse's story…

"One of my friends was on duty in casualty and I was in the neurosurgical ward. We had decided that we would definitely go out that night. My friend had bought a new pair of white jeans and was determined to wear them to some social event.

My ward was busy and we had a number of army personnel as some of our patients were injured soldiers. One of them was extremely ill; he had been shot in the head and back with a particular type of ammunition which caused extreme damage inside the body. He was 22 years old and his parents were sitting with him, having travelled across from England to be with their only son. He was very ill and we, and they, knew that the end was near.

Also in the ward we had a patient who had come to us from a foreign shipping trawler and who had sustained a head injury in a fall from a mast. He was covered from head to toe in tattoos and it provided a degree of light relief from the weighty demands of the ward when he would ask which tattoo we would use to give his injection that day. He spoke very little English and we all tried to ensure that he felt content during his stay with us. Another gentleman was totally in awe of the fact that he had a titanium plate inserted in his skull. He told everyone in the vicinity that part of his skull was now the same material that was used in air force jets.

Crowd invades RVH

Stormy scenes occurred at Belfast's Royal Victoria Hospital yesterday when a crowd, mostly of young girls, invaded the casualty department.

Trouble erupted when the mob learned that a number of Maze prisoners had been brought in for treatment for cuts and bruises.

About 200 people forced their way into the department and flung themselves on police and soldiers guarding the prisoners.

For a time there was a struggle, fists flying, and at one stage the crowd attempted to drag a prisoner from a trolley on which he was lying before treatment.

Word began to filter down that something was wrong in Long Kesh. It transpired that there had been a fire and those with injuries were being ferried to the Royal. Casualty was put on alert.

Our unit was quiet as our patients required a calm environment. Though many were acutely ill and some others dying, the ward was tranquil. Staff were busy, relatives were sitting with their loved ones and the foreign sailor was joking with one of the nurses about the injection.

But then things changed as reports from casualty suggested that people were being admitted with burn injuries. Other reports suggested that some were dead on arrival, police and army were everywhere, sirens began to wail continuously and friends and relatives of prisoners were arriving in a very anxious state.

I was walking toward the main doors when I heard an almighty racket and suddenly people appeared from nowhere, running about in a highly emotional state. These were folks arriving to look for relatives they thought were dead or injured in the fire at Long Kesh and, not finding them in casualty, were setting off in search of them. The place became chaotic – equipment was knocked over

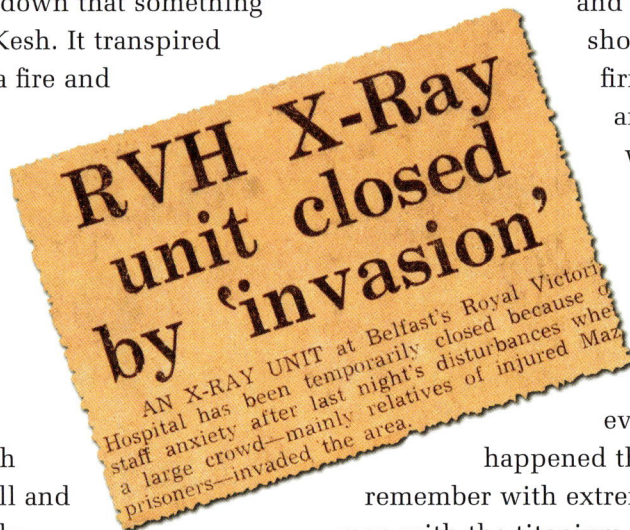

RVH X-Ray unit closed by 'invasion'

AN X-RAY UNIT at Belfast's Royal Victory Hospital has been temporarily closed because o staff anxiety after last night's disturbances whe a large crowd—mainly relatives of injured Maz prisoners—invaded the area.

and people were shouting. I was taken firmly by the collar and told quite clearly what would happen to me if I didn't tell them where their relative had been taken. Even today, I choose not to speak of everything that happened that day. What I do remember with extreme pain is that the man with the titanium plate became frozen with fear, the sailor stopped joking and the soldier died.

We didn't go out that night, but we did the following week. We walked down the Falls Road towards the Grosvenor and suddenly a gun battle erupted.

Shouts of 'Get down! Get down!' rang in our ears.

We did, spreadeagled on the ground, so both sides could see we posed no danger. After about two or three minutes of heavy firing, we were still lying on the ground and my friend turned to me and said: 'You know what? My white jeans are going to get ruined.'

With bullets whizzing past and a full on gun battle in progress, worrying about new jeans demonstrated the sort of denial so frequently exhibited during those years. **"**

A serious dressing down

"Whilst working as a staff nurse at Musgrave Park surgical ward in 1984-85, there was a well known, formidable but well-respected Nursing Officer.

We had a patient who had inadvertently triggered a car bomb he was attempting to plant and was injured in the ensuing explosion. He had severe burns on the back of his body and was being nursed lying on his front with a cage over his back. He had a police guard which the police decided to remove as the man was so severely injured and was on very strong intravenous pain relief.

As I was going off duty one evening about nine o'clock, three men walked past me in the corridor leading from the ward. They were walking three abreast very close to each other and the one in the middle was wearing a track suit and looked somewhat the worse for wear.

The two outside men had raincoats draped over their arms.

It occurred to me that this might be our burned bomber but I had not seen his face properly and I had not been directly looking after him in the previous few days. The two men on the outside bid me good evening as they passed and when I turned round I could see that the feet of the man in the middle were barely touching the ground. I was suspicious so immediately retraced my steps back up to the ward, checked his cubicle. He was gone. I immediately alerted the ward staff and security and didn't get home till quite late that night.

The next morning I was summoned by the Nursing Officer who demanded to know why I hadn't challenged the men. After a serious dressing down, I suggested that they may have had guns and I didn't think it the right thing to do. She thanked me for my written statement and suggested that I have an extra 15 minutes' tea break. What a lady!**"**

Trauma

"When asked to remove a severed leg I was completely taken aback, not only having to do it, but by how heavy and awkward an amputated limb could be."

First-year Student Nurse

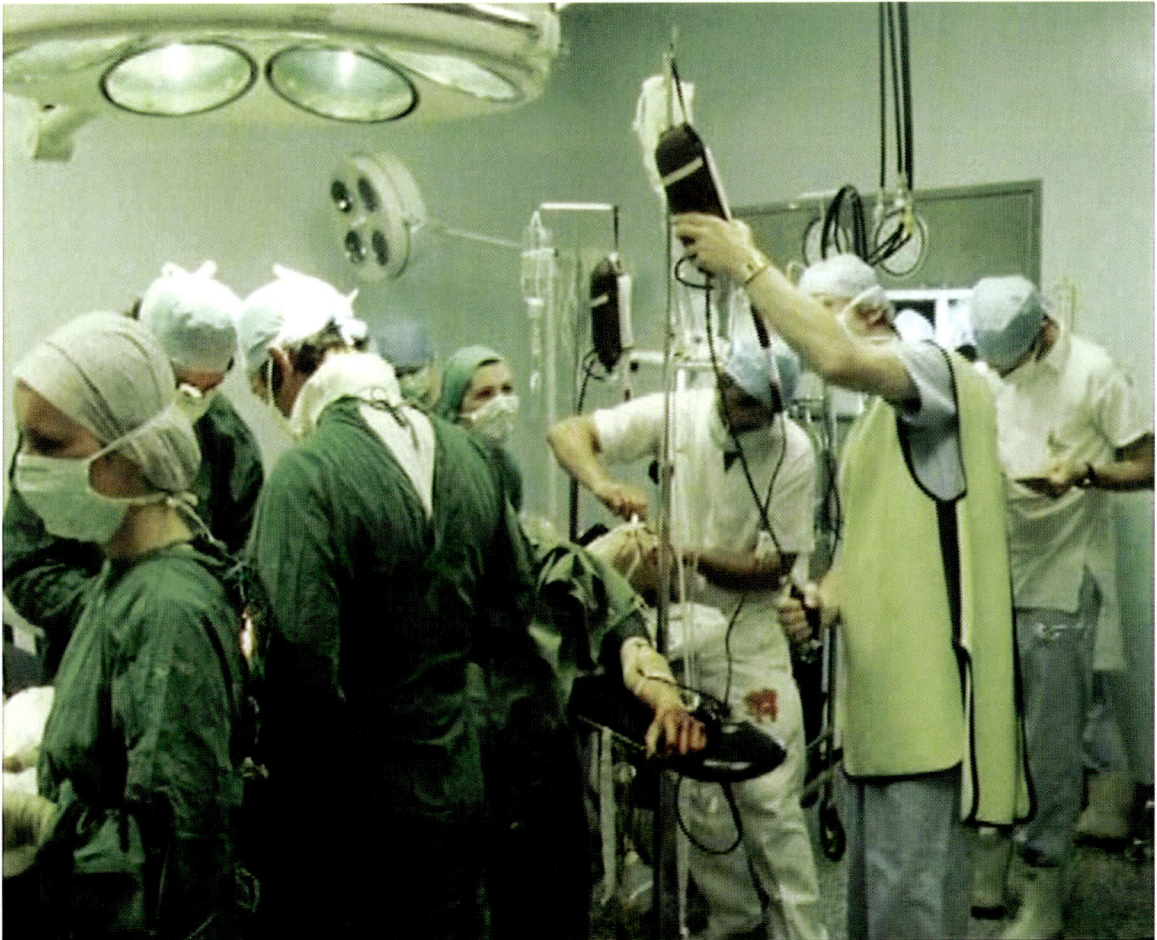

© BBC

115

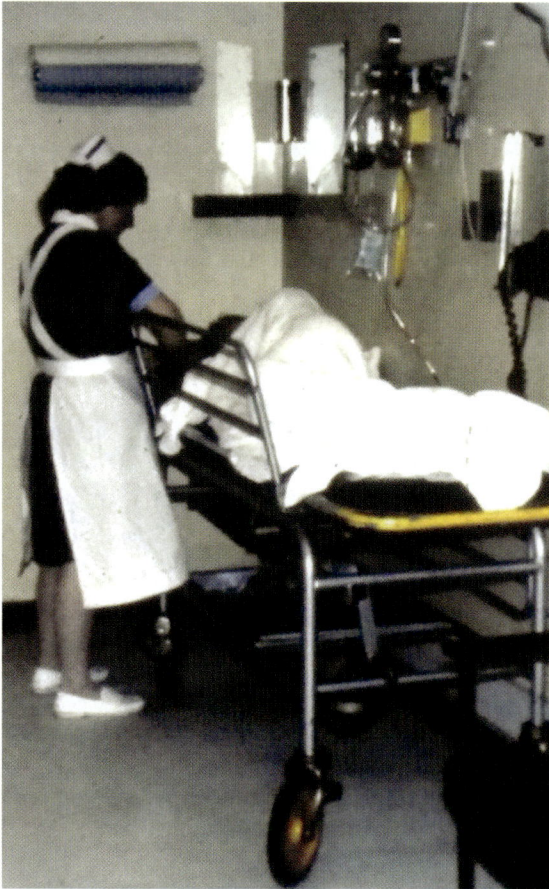
Casualty major – injury cubicle

Those who had chosen to develop their careers in these areas had decades of experience and managing casualties wounded from bomb or bullet became automatic. On reflection a theatre nurse recounted how for her:

"The abnormal became the normal and I did not always realise how exposure to such trauma would affect newcomers to theatre."
Altnagelvin Staff Nurse

Accident and emergency departments, theatre units and specialist units, such as intensive care, neurosurgery and burns, all cared for many trauma victims.

Wherever and whenever violence erupted across the province, the injured were brought to the nearest casualty for immediate assessment. Following major incidents, victims who had been killed were also often brought to casualty. This was traumatic for all staff involved.

Major emergency and trauma units

Nurses who worked in the acute service areas, including accident and emergency and theatres, still have disturbed memories. All recounted unexpected flashbacks evoked by certain sights, smells and taste.

As one theatre nurse remarked "I remember the smell of dirt, gunpowder, dried blood and burnt flesh." Another accident and emergency nurse recalled: "It was a long time before I could look at raw meat."

All casualties were treated according to the severity of their injury. The Royal Victoria Hospital (RVH) in Belfast was the regional trauma centre with all the recognised facilities for intensive care, neurosurgery, orthopaedics and cardiac surgery. Throughout the Troubles patients were either stabilised in a local hospital or flown directly to the RVH in Belfast.

Key departments became skilled at initiating disaster plans at a moment's notice. Mr Rutherford, consultant A&E doctor at the RVH, re-designed and developed a disaster plan that became a template for national use.

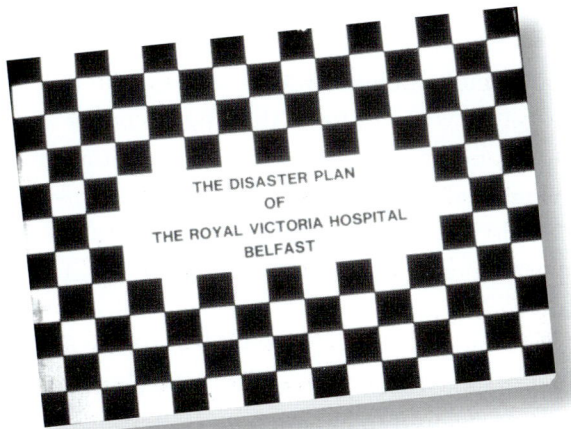
Front cover of RVH Disaster Plan

The Royal's major incident plan

The Royal Victoria Hospital (RVH), in accordance with Department of Health policy, had a major incident plan for implementation in the event of a major disaster. However as Miss Robb, matron of the RVH recalls, Mr Rutherford, the accident and emergency consultant, reviewed and radically changed this disaster plan to emphasise that all staff continued, as far as possible, doing what for them was routine.

The admission form was redesigned so that less but important information could be written up quickly. A new command and communication system was put in place. As this was before the days of mobile phones and small switchboard systems could easily become jammed by too many calls, it was important to contact all key personnel quickly, either by phone or by paging. A fan-shaped communication system was developed whereby the telephonist contacted a named person who then contacted someone else in the chain and so on. "Red phones" which had a direct line out avoiding switchboard, were introduced to certain departments including nursing administration. This system also had built into it a "double check" to ensure that all key personnel were informed.

Following a bomb explosion, patients often arrived at the same time and in large numbers. It was important that all injured were quickly sorted, with those most injured receiving immediate treatment. This triage of patients required skilled doctors and nurses using back-up from other departments so that those patients who needed immediate surgery were admitted quickly. In the first three years of its development, the disaster plan was invoked 48 times for bombings and 15 times for rioting. The plan was adapted by many hospitals across the UK.

"We had a disaster plan. It worked well on the day of the bomb… we were congratulated on our records."
Sister, Erne Hospital, Enniskillen

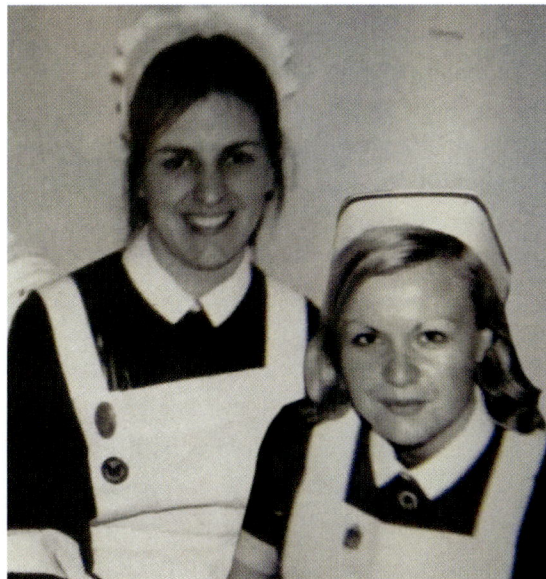
Casualty sister and staff nurse

Fall from a lookout tower

A Craigavon casualty nurse remembers…

"It was a soldier who had been shot dead while he was at the top of a high lookout tower. He dropped to the ground and obviously landed on his feet.

In casualty we had to undress patients who were dead to identify them, record their injuries and attempt to certify cause of death. I saw his lifeless face; he was in his early twenties, close to my own age.

I felt unnerved as he had dark hair and swarthy skin, and resembled my brother, except his eyes didn't sparkle with devilment and his pupils were fixed and dilated.

I felt relieved to be at the foot end of the body and began to unlace his boots. I could hear and feel the crepitus of his bones, crunching and crackling. His legs were in smithereens. When I loosened the laces his feet swung and turned back-to-front, his toes facing their opposite anatomical position. It reminded me of a toy action man figure that I'd seen children play with. I knew if I tried to yank his boots off that his feet would be left dangling.

'I can't do this,' I said in a panic. I'd never experienced anything like this before. A senior doctor came to my aid, but he was also visibly shocked. He re-tied the bootlaces and bound the ankles together, each acting as splint for the other.

Sometimes nurses are seen, and expected, 'to get on with it'. Later that night I broke down and apologised to the same doctor for being weak. I will never forget his response. He said: 'Don't apologise for crying. It's a sign you care. I would think less of you if you didn't react.'

I learned a lesson that night and was never again ashamed to shed a tear. I often slipped into the sluice room to dry my eyes and met colleagues who were there for the same reason."

Murder triangle

"In the early days those of us who worked as students in the emergency and intensive care units of the Mater Hospital quickly became experienced clinical practitioners even though we were only at the beginning of our careers.

We didn't have 'trolley waits', bed managers or targets or directors of anything. As the security situation changed so too did the management of trauma victims. Better systems were developed and more resources became available. Those were the days, in the early 1970s, before triage; working in an A&E department in the area of the city known as 'murder triangle'. At night, working with three nurses and one junior doctor, we developed our own system for dealing with the sudden arrival of 30 victims from a bombed pub.

Improvised 'standard operating procedures' were employed to deal with an emergency department full of victims of one atrocity or another, with the mix of life-threatening injuries and the walking wounded. Our medically-based model of nurse training stood us in good stead in those days. Maybe we were the forerunners of nurse practitioners and the triage system. Circumstances often resulted in the blurring of roles between doctors and nurses as we did our best in some awful situations.

My memories are of the unsure junior house officer dealing with his first gunshot wound and of the camaraderie between the young doctors and nurses, dealing on a daily basis with the traumatic scenes of carnage which were North Belfast in the 1970s. Often the junior doctors, seeing trauma for the first time, relied on the advice and sometimes intervention of an experienced staff nurse.

I look back on those early days with a mixture of terrible sadness at the unnecessary loss of young lives, and pride to have worked in such a unique place with many exceptional nurses and doctors. Many lifelong friendships were forged in those days. **"**

Theatre nursing

Theatre staff became adept at interrupting planned surgical lists to set up for trauma casualties. Speed was of the essence and it was not unknown for a casualty to be undergoing surgery within 15 minutes of injury.

Nurses who worked in theatre units in all hospitals described how they had to be prepared for the unexpected.

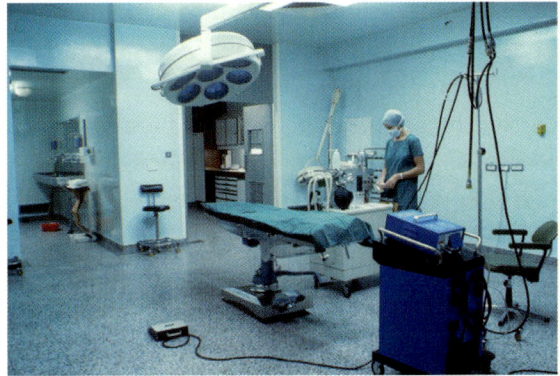

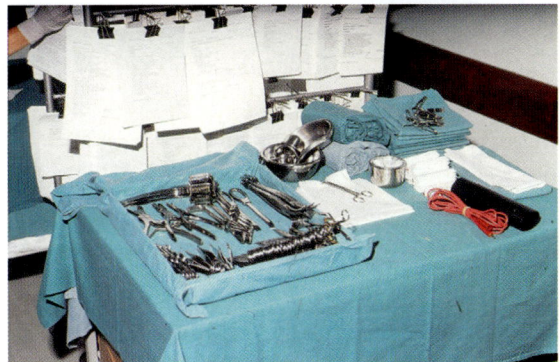

Trauma - general theatre, 1970s

A theatre sister's story

"It is no longer possible to recall precise details of every disaster, as all now seem to fuse together in the mind and memory. Some are still mentioned today in the news, as relatives seek information, inquiry or 'closure'. With each so-named atrocity, memories return.

When asked for my first recollection, I'd say the smell. Following a bombing this was a mixture of explosive and injured flesh. Patients sent to theatre as soon as possible were often wearing the remains of their clothes, torn and full of dust. Clothing removed in A&E would be put in a plastic bag on the trolley. Examining these bags was difficult. Finding personal items such as pension books, car and house keys, wallets with photographs, everyday things that are carried by all, were sometimes barely recognisable. Often, when the identity of patients was not known, they were labelled 'A, B, C' and so on in order of admission. I remember passing a piece of jewellery to a member of admin staff outside the theatre window, to be taken to relatives as a means of patient identification.

There were other difficulties with clothing. If the injured patient was a suspected terrorist, clothes were to be retained for forensic examination. On one occasion, relatives managed to arrive at the entrance lobby to theatres, though not through the air-lock doors. They banged on the windows, shouting loudly and begging for the clothes. The patient was a boy of about 17 years, who did not survive. It was hard to listen to his mother's crying, without feeling sympathy for all who found themselves in these awful situations.

Some injuries will never be forgotten, nor the sight of a very senior surgeon with tears in his eyes. We comforted and supported each other, fortunate that most of us had worked together for years and the team spirit and trust helped us to keep going as did our 'nursing humour' with each other, which was not always polite!

I shared the theatre nursing admin duties with two colleagues. At the start of the Troubles, many staff, on hearing bad news, would come on duty voluntarily. It became necessary to form an on-call rota of the

three of us, as routine surgical lists had to resume as soon as possible. Only the necessary number of staff were called, ensuring that those not required did not feel guilty, and were then available for routine duties next day. Saturday evening was a frequent disaster time. When on call, it was a relief to wake on Sunday morning and think: 'I wasn't called.'

Writing about all this makes these events seem quite recent, instead of almost 40 years ago. I hope that these dark days will never be repeated.**"**

She never flinched

A theatre staff nurse recalls…

"When bomb casualties arrived in theatre direct from casualty, their wounds were often grossly contaminated. Clothes were usually badly torn and covered in thick white dust from collapsed masonry. Brick dust blasted into deep wounds was a perfect recipe for gas gangrene and other deadly infections.

Before patients could be allowed into a sterile operating theatre, the worst of the debris had to be washed off. But that couldn't happen until the patient was anaesthetised. Clothing would then be cut off in the anaesthetic room, and the patient's body decontaminated with scrubbing brushes and large basins of disinfectant.

One evening in 1975 this procedure was under way, observed by a student nurse on night duty. If anyone qualified for the description "a slip of a girl" it was she. Small and slight, not long since she had been a schoolgirl. Students then spent only six weeks in theatre during training, just enough to acclimatise.

During removal of the bomb victim's trousers, his lower right leg flopped where his knee used to be, and then dangled freely. It was now attached to his thigh by only a mass of shattered bone and shredded muscle. I gave the student an unobtrusive neutral glance, in case she should be prone to fainting.

She never flinched. I never saw one that did flinch."

Respiratory and intensive care unit

The respiratory care centre at the Royal Victoria Hospital was set up in 1959 and in 1969 developed in size and role as a newly built 12-bed unit, the respiratory and intensive care unit, commonly referred to as RICU. The unit comprised six single wards and a six-bed open ward, and there was also a hyperbaric oxygen chamber.

The unit was later extended and upgraded to include two additional bed spaces making it one of the largest units in the UK. Patients were nursed "one to one" (one nurse to one patient). The unit was built close to casualty, which meant that trauma patients could be transferred quickly to the unit, and consultant anaesthetists were readily accessible to provide expert respiratory care to any casualty.

The benefit of such close proximity was fully realised during major incidents. When the Troubles broke out, RICU was one of the wards at the front line of treating casualties severely damaged by bombs, bullets and punishment beatings. Many of these injuries were life-threatening.

Casualties treated included civilians, security personnel and paramilitaries. When either of the latter were patients, a security guard sat at the entrance to the ward. On one occasion gunmen shot dead a policeman on duty at the ward entrance. Following the attack, this entrance was made more secure and strengthened with bullet-proof glass.

Needless to say, there was an almost permanent presence of armed policemen or soldiers at the entrance to RICU and the shooting at the ward door added to the stress of all staff.

The year 1972 is recognised as the worst year of the Troubles because of the high number of deaths and casualties. This was a year of intense bombing which killed and injured many civilians. One of the sisters in RICU noted that, of the patients cared for that year, 76 had gunshot wounds and 16 were the victims of bomb explosions. For the same period, casualty had 493 gunshot wounds and 371 admissions due to blast injury or assault.

The following stories are recounted by nurses who worked at different times in RICU...

Nursing in intensive care

"I was very aware of the start of the Troubles but especially the arrival of the British army, as my niece was born on 14 August 1969. My sister was sent home early after the birth because there was trouble in Belfast.

The new RICU was nearing completion. It fully opened in early 1970 with six single rooms and a large area for six bed spaces. Little did we realise how often all these would be fully occupied.

The numbers admitted due to the Troubles began slowly and the first large disaster I remember was when a bomb exploded in the Abercorn Cafe in Belfast. It was a quiet Saturday afternoon. The casualties were many and some had horrendous injuries. Two sisters were admitted, one having lost both legs and an arm and the other both legs. A man who was due to be married in a few weeks had lost both legs and a lady was admitted with the leg of a chair lodged through her leg. There were many more.

This was the first time I and many of my colleagues had seen such injuries. We had to learn quickly how to tell these patients the extent of their injuries, answering their questions with honesty and compassion.

I remember a peaceful Sunday afternoon when I was first asked, 'When will the pain go away and my legs heal?' The answer, sadly, was: 'You have lost both legs.' I spent a long time with the patient, a young woman, that day. These circumstances made the workload unpredictable and stressful, but rewarding.

Many incidents are crowding into my head. The young soldier who appeared unconscious, having been shot in the head, until his commanding officer came to visit and spoke to him. The soldier then struggled to get his hand to his head to salute.

The relatives waiting to see their loved ones were of all political persuasions but comforting each other. This helped us as nurses not to think of who they were, but all as anxious relatives together. There were many Belfast people who volunteered to look after the army families, who were in an alien country. They took them to their homes and to the shops. The relatives had accommodation in the hospital.

I remember many of the people who I nursed but one of them presented a particular challenge. A soldier had been caught in an explosion in Crossmaglen, where a colleague was killed and a

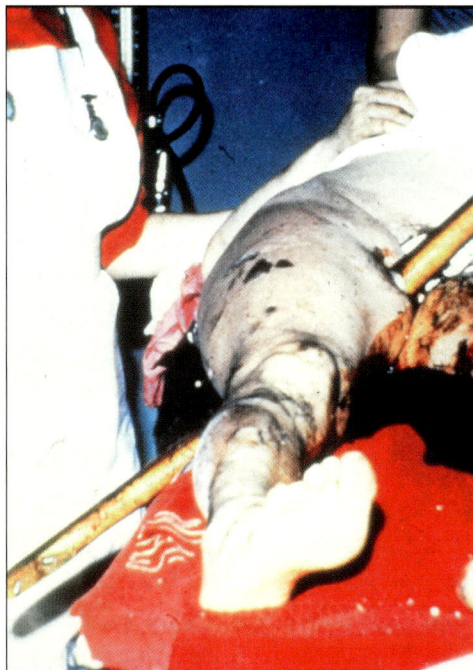
Bomb injury

policeman blinded. Derek had had half of his face blown away. He was admitted to RICU with his head completely bandaged. He also had a bad leg injury. He required to be ventilated. His wife, we discovered, was 37 weeks pregnant with her second child, past the time when she could officially travel by air. Derek's condition was such that it was important for her to come from Germany. With a lot of persuasion from the medical and nursing staff the red tape was cut and she duly arrived.

In spite of Derek's terrible injuries her first words were 'That is my Derek'. Three weeks later I was privileged to be with her in the Royal Maternity Hospital when she gave birth to a lovely baby girl. I was able to tell Derek he had a second daughter. I have been able to stay friends with the family but sadly Derek died of cancer a couple of years ago having lived a very restricted life for 30 years. As nurses we are not often able to follow a patient for that length of time.

Some children were caught in the bombs and crossfire and had to be admitted to the adult unit. This required us to extend our knowledge and redesign equipment to treat them. This was a time of dreadful loss and tragedy, and the full realisation of man's inhumanity to man. But there were many positives too. Huge advances were made in treating casualties very soon after their initial injuries. Head injuries, either from gunshot or blast, were treated with relaxation and artificial respiration to reduce cerebral oedema. Chest injuries were usually caused by blast and treated, again, by relaxation and ventilation. Reducing blood loss when limbs were blown off was essential as this was a

cause of high mortality. This type of injury has been seen in Iraq and Afghanistan where early treatment is imperative, as we soon came to realise in Belfast all those years ago.

The experience gained by nursing and medical staff was huge. The junior nurses, many in their first year, benefitted from the closeness of the trained staff who were always available to answer queries and help the juniors gain knowledge and confidence. I won a scholarship to the US in 1973 where I gave several talks and presented what became known as 'My war pictures'. My salary was low in comparison to US rates so I was paid $50 for each talk.

There was unfortunately a high mortality rate because of the severe nature of the injuries to young, fit males in the main. Transplantation of kidneys was at an early stage of development. I spent a great deal of time with relatives and I came to know them very well. I was frequently able to talk to them about donation of their loved one's kidneys, with great effect. In many instances the transplant was successful. These kidneys went all over Europe and it gave the relatives some comfort to know the death of their loved ones was not entirely in vain.

The positive thing I remember most was the great relationship amongst the staff, medical, nursing and ancillary workers. These included ward clerks, orderlies, and domestics. We knew each other so well. I think about the staff nurse whose husband was a policeman, the domestic who was concerned about her grandson and the company he was keeping, and the nurse whose children's school had been evacuated

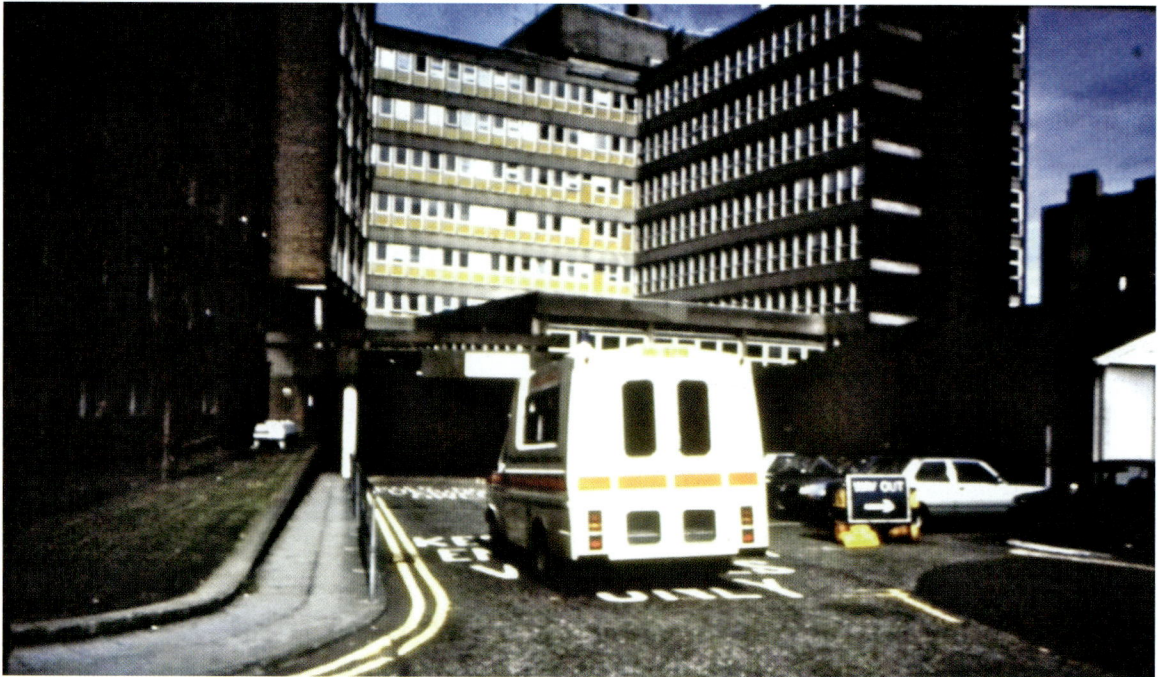

A&E Ambulance RVH, 1970s

because of a bomb. They now had lessons with their coats kept under their desks. This had a traumatic effect on the children. These people all needed time to talk and this we would do when having a break. We did, however, have a social life too. When we could, we would arrange, often at short notice, a meal out together. Sometimes though, it had to be cancelled due to incidents requiring the full staff on duty.

For me personally, it was in 1974 that I met my husband. When I hear of shooting or bombs in any country my mind goes back to my days in Northern Ireland because one can never forget that time. The experience has obviously affected my whole life and especially shaped my later nursing career. I am pleased to say that I still return to Northern Ireland to see family and friends and have lovely holidays. It is certainly a different place today. **"**

The bent nail

"My only involvement in a major incident was while I was on an intensive care placement in Craigavon Hospital.

I had worked a long day and was off at 9pm. I was having tea in the nurses' home where I stayed during my three-year training. I heard ambulance after ambulance go past to the hospital. I used the internal phone to call A&E offering to help and was told to come and bring any staff that were in the home with me. This was around Christmas and New Year celebrations and apparently a bomb had gone off in a bar/night club injuring many people.

When I arrived in A&E the casualties had started to arrive and were being admitted and identified by numbers as they came in. Several other students and I stood waiting to be assigned to a patient. I remember the nurse just in front of me being asked to stay with a man who seemed to have had his abdomen blown off exposing his intestines. I remember the doctor examining him and asking the nurse to get him morphine for pain and to stay with the man as nothing more could be done. So the nurse stayed with him until he died. I remember thinking that I was glad I wasn't the one asked.

I was assigned a 19-year-old man who seemed okay except he could not bend his right leg. He was in a wheel chair and after being examined I was to stay with him and bring him to X-ray, wait, and then return him and the X-ray to A&E. I spoke to the young man and he said he was in the club with his friend enjoying themselves when, suddenly without warning, everything blew up.

He could not understand why his leg couldn't move. He had no pain and apart from a few scratches from flying glass he didn't seem to be seriously injured. He was concerned about his friend and others he was with, and was both orientated and talking freely.

After some time waiting he finally had the X-ray and, looking at it, I could not believe what I saw. Right inside his bone was a six-inch nail which was bent in the middle causing his knee to lie at a 90° angle. I wondered how a nail could have placed itself inside the bone both above and below the knee and bend at right angles.

We arrived back at A&E and waited again. As my patient was one of the 'walking wounded' with no obvious life-threatening injury, we waited for about another hour. When he was seen again, the doctor told him he needed to go to theatre to have the nail removed. I stayed with him in theatre and scrubbed up when he had surgery at about 2.30am.

Unfortunately things were not as simple as first thought and he developed circulatory problems and began bleeding. The surgeons took the decision to amputate his leg just above the knee. I had to hold the leg while they removed it. After the operation I continued with the patient into recovery and performed observations until about 5am. When an ICU bed became available I transferred him. I continued until 6.30am when Sister told me to get some breakfast before my day shift started at 7.30am.

After breakfast, a shower and a change of clothes I returned to my normal placement in ICU and to my patient at 7.30am. I remember looking after this young man and being there when he awoke a few hours later. He was told they had amputated his leg. In the next bed beside him was his friend who, believe it or not, had also had his left leg amputated, just above the knee.

The next few days I was performing care as usual except there were lots of relatives, friends and media attention. As students we were told not to answer any questions from media but to refer all queries and enquiries to sister or the person in charge.

I remember about a week or so later the two young people were joking that they'd only have to buy one pair of shoes between them, he getting the left shoe and the other the right. 🙰

Memories of RICU

The door of the intensive care unit was kept locked and guarded inside by two soldiers as there were security force patients in the unit. One evening, two men wearing white doctors' coats came to the door.

When one of the soldiers on guard opened it, the men fired their guns, then escaped via a convenient exit to the main road. The sister on duty, with a student nurse, immediately ran to the door and attended the wounded soldier without any thought for their own safety. Sadly, that young soldier died. The sister was later awarded the MBE.

On another occasion a young soldier was admitted to the unit with an extremely damaged face after an explosive device had blown up in front of him. The plastic surgeons did what they could but he ended up totally unlike his previous good-looking self. I often wondered what it must have been like for him, returning home to face his family and friends with his appearance so changed. Some years later I met him in England, and I was filled with admiration for his personal courage as he continued to enjoy life.**

Neurosurgery

"I remember one policeman with a head injury due to the propellers of a helicopter hitting him on the head. He couldn't speak but we soon discovered he could sing."
Royal Victoria Hospital Student Nurse

The RVH had a dedicated neurosurgery ward and theatre. During the Troubles the staff developed skills in the management of serious head injuries. The use of a titanium plate to cover skull defects was first developed by two RVH consultants.

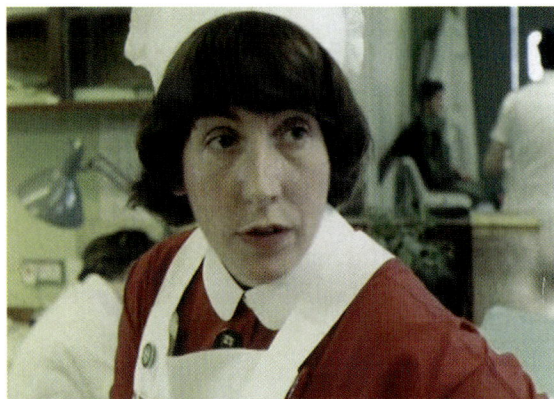
Neurosurgery Sister

Titanium cranioplasty

A neurosurgery sister describes the procedure and recalls the case of a police officer with a head injury…

Before 1974, skull defects were repaired using bone grafts taken from the iliac crest or moulds made from acrylic material. These were roughly shaped to cover the damaged section of the skull. The results however were often uneven, giving a 'bumpy' appearance and plates often had to be removed because of infection.

The escalation of violence at this time resulted in many more extensive head wounds. The resultant skull defects were much larger and more difficult to repair using the conventional methods. Bomb blast injuries and high-velocity bullet injuries shattered the skull leaving defects of up to 6cm × 4cm in some cases.

Consultant Neurosurgeon Derek Gordon and Consultant Dental Surgeon George Blair worked together to find a more suitable substance than bone or acrylic. Titanium – the metal used in the construction of spacecraft and Concorde wings at that time – was used because of its great strength and superb ability to be shaped to the exact contour of the patient's head.

An impression of the patient's head was taken with the same material that dentists use for taking teeth impressions. From this a plaster cast was made and then a model of the patient's head showing the damaged section from which the plate was to be precisely fashioned. A flap of skin was cut over the damaged area of the skull to allow access to the bone beneath.

The plate was fastened into place with tiny titanium screws, which also have to be made to the exact thickness of the patient's skull. Then the skin flap is sewn down again and the hair grows back on it very quickly.

Over the years and with advancements such as computer technology, the technique has been modified and improved. It is widely used to treat patients with defects resulting

from congenital malformations, head trauma and to replace bone that has to be removed because of disease or infection.. "

One of her patients was Harry, aged 28 years...

A victim of the Ulster Polytechnic bomb, November 1983[1]

Harry was admitted to the A&E department of the Royal Victoria Hospital, on Friday 4 November 1983. A married man with two young children, he was a sergeant in the RUC. Harry had sustained multiple injuries in a bomb explosion 30 minutes earlier. This had occurred in the Ulster Polytechnic where he and some of his colleagues were attending lectures to gain a certificate in Police Studies.

Harry's wife Mary was informed of his injuries, and came to his bedside in the intensive care unit (ICU). Before her marriage she had been a nurse in our hospital, but since the birth of her children she had not worked. In the civil disturbances in Northern Ireland, policemen's wives have to live with the possibility that their husbands may be injured or killed. They cope by pushing the thought to the back of their minds, and live each day as it comes.

Earlier that morning Harry had kissed Mary and the children as he left the house to attend the polytechnic. Mary did not realise then that it would be the last voluntary kiss she would receive from her husband. She expected him home for his evening meal; she could not have expected to be sitting by his bedside in an ICU. True, Mary was a nurse and had been used to nursing critically ill patients. She had some idea of what to expect when

---

[1]RVH League of Nurses, No 37, April 1986

it came to Harry's appearance. Of course the situation is very different when that critically ill patient is a very close relative.

Transfer to the neurosurgical unit

After four weeks in ICU, Harry was transferred to the neurosurgical unit for further management. He seemed to regress rather than improve. He would cry out frequently and appear to be in pain. He would intermittently draw his knees up to his chest and would constantly clench his teeth. He would pull his right ear and grimace. He would hit out at the nurses and his wife, and resented any interference. No physical reason was found to cause this obvious agitation and manic behaviour.

This was an extremely frustrating time for Harry's wife and the nursing staff; we all felt so helpless because nothing seemed to settle him. Initially treatment with antidepressants seemed to help.

His wife visited him for long periods daily, and we involved her in his nursing care. She felt she was doing something positive to help him, and he certainly seemed to be calmer when she was there.

Mary felt it important for the children to visit their father, in spite of some opposition from the rest of the family. They were bewildered at first, and naturally could not understand why Daddy 'would not speak' to them. However they soon started to talk, and the children would draw little pictures for Harry's room. Naturally a lot of Mary's time was taken up with visiting Harry. The children seemed to accept this. Mary explained to them that she couldn't devote

as much time to them, as she had to help the nurses to look after their father when he was sick. She did, however, take them on frequent outings to compensate for her absence on other occasions.

The security wing of the ward

Harry was always nursed in the security wing of our ward, except for visits to radiology or physiotherapy. Patients were termed 'security' if they were members of the police force, Ulster Defence Regiment, British army, prison service, judiciary, or if they were politicians or indeed terrorists.

For almost 16 years Northern Ireland has suffered from what the news media call 'urban guerrilla warfare'. Our hospital, which has a full range of surgical and medical specialties for the province, is situated in the middle of one of the troubled areas of Belfast. For this reason members of the security forces admitted to the hospital are vulnerable to attempts on their lives. Since 1969 therefore, injured or ill security personnel have been under guard while in the hospital.

Following attempts on their lives by terrorists in 1982, the British government ruled that these patients must be guarded in secure areas, one of which exists in our unit. The patients are nursed in single rooms, two rooms in ward 40, and three in ward 39. Cameras monitor activity on the staircase and outside two sets of bulletproof doors. Police guards inside the secure area observe the closed-circuit television screens. Entry to the rooms is gained by summoning the guard on the intercom.

This system works well, provided the patient is not too ill. If the patient requires frequent nursing care or is restless or confused, we find it necessary for a nurse to remain in constant attendance. To avoid conflict, we try to ensure that patients from opposing factions are not nursed in adjoining rooms. Flare-ups can arise between sets of relatives, or between guards and relatives. When this happens, the senior nurse has to mediate between the two to resolve problems before the rest of the ward is disrupted. In the absence of security patients, these rooms can be used for ordinary patients.

Problems are encountered when an ordinary patient has to be nursed in the secure area, due to shortage of beds. Some patients accept the situation; but there are also those who object, chiefly because they are frightened. A solution has to be reached which is acceptable to the patient and nursing and medical staff. This can involve transfer of another patient to another ward in the hospital.

The existence of a security area in an acute neurosurgical unit certainly adds to the nurse's workload. It is, however, the best method to date that we have to protect these men when they are receiving specialised treatment in the hospital. Nursing staff do not object to working in the area, and its existence is discussed with them at interview. Immediate action must always be taken to resolve any problems that arise. In this respect we are fortunate to have good liaison with the local police station.

Towards the end of May 1984 Harry's condition deteriorated. It was now obvious that he was not going to recover. Mary had been gradually prepared for this. She continued to involve herself in his care. She was with him when he became comatose and died peacefully on 12 August 1984, nine months after the explosion. He was the 200th member of the RUC to die in Northern Ireland as a result of the civil disturbances. **"**

A love of poetry

"I speciallied in ward 21, then neurosurgery, at the Royal Victoria Hospital. One of my patients was a policeman shot during the Troubles.

Someone knocked on his door and he opened his upstairs window and looked out to see who it was. He was shot in the head. His brain was badly damaged.

I always loved poetry and so did the patient and his wife. I always associate him with the 'Lake Isle of Innisfree' by WB Yeats. 'I will arise and go now, and go to Innisfree...' I would say one line of the poem and he would say the following line, even with his severe brain injuries.

I never fail to read that poem without thinking of him and it brings a lump to my throat. He was still in ward 21 when I moved on to my next ward and I often wonder how things went for him and his wife. **"**

No labels

"I was on night duty and living in the Towers. One day I was awakened by the noise of gunshots, then sirens of police cars, fire brigade and ambulances.

That night I went to work on ward 21 (neurosurgery). A travelling salesman who had been driving round the roundabout was caught in the crossfire of a gun battle between the IRA and the army. That night he was a patient on the ward. This man had been paralysed by a bullet. He would never walk again.

On another occasion I remember one of the consultant surgeons being hijacked on the Falls Road. His car was stolen and he was just left on the street.

Ward 21 holds many memories for me. British soldiers, policemen, civilians, Irish republicans, firemen and taxi drivers were all patients at one time or another, often with severe injuries. All were cared for tenderly and professionally. No labels, other than 'injured', 'post-operative' or 'long stay'. There were soldiers guarding on this ward at all times.

We used to have fun with these boys and they would actually help us lift patients and turn them. No wonder we all have back problems. Some romances started between nurses and soldiers. Some nurses married policemen they had nursed.

On another surgical ward, I nursed well-known prisoners whose names will go down in the history of the Troubles.

Their photographs can be seen in accounts of the history of hunger strikers and such like. It was difficult at times, but you had to treat everyone the same. I did – you had to guard your heart from bitterness and anger.**"**

Burn injuries

A Staff Nurse seconded to the Ulster Hospital remembers…

"During my 18 years at the Royal Victoria Hospital, I, like many others, nursed victims of the Troubles: the Abercorn, McGurk's Bar, La Mon Hotel and the Dunmurry train, to name a few. During that time clinical treatments and practices changed.

I remember the very first time I had to nurse two patients with serious burns. They were injured while making explosives. Both were in their early twenties and had sustained extensive full-thickness burns to 80% of their bodies.

This was in the early 1970s, and there was no specialist burns unit, nor were there any experienced nurses trained in caring for the patient with burns. The patients were nursed in a side room and lay on green sterile towels. The wounds were left exposed. With such extensive burns, it was recognised that all we could do was ensure the patients were kept as comfortable as possible.

In 1977-78 I undertook a specialist course in burns and plastic surgery. I was seconded to work in the Ulster Hospital to care for a number of patients admitted with severe burns following the La Mon bombing. By this stage, the treatment for full-thickness burns was early excision and grafting, and all wounds were dressed using Flamazine cream. A far cry from when I nursed my first burns patient. Burns victims require a high intensity of nursing care. It was not easy to care for these patients in an open ward, but the Ulster Hospital managed extremely well.

A number of patients had very severe burns which required many operations, long months in recovery and convalescence. When patients have severe burns they wake up every day and the scars are still there. Many from La Mon had facial and hand scars, obvious to everyone they met.

In 1979, a much-needed burns unit was commissioned which provided excellent accommodation and care for patients with burns. A dedicated multidisciplinary team, led by a consultant plastic surgeon developed the service and changed practices in the care and treatment of burns.

Having a dedicated theatre meant patients could have surgery earlier while experienced nursing staff, dedicated physiotherapy, occupational therapy, dietetics and social services all contributed to better experiences and outcomes. Improved pain relief was used for dressing changes. Skin taken for grafting was meshed to spread it further and prevent a haematoma occurring under the skin graft. Pressure garments were fitted to reduce or prevent scarring and contractures.

Grateful Nursing Mirror thanks. 6·11·80

OUTGOING Rcn President Eirlys Rees paid tribute to the nurses of Northern Ireland.

"Many injured victims of terrorism will have cause to be grateful to the nursing service of Northern Ireland, which has continued to function, often under considerable strain, throughout the last 10 years.

"These victims — Protestant and Catholic alike — have been the beneficiaries of an ethical principle that holds there are no frontiers and no political or religious constraints in tending the sick."

She supported the Rcn's policy of no industrial action. "I do not regard this as outmoded and unthinking pacifism. I prefer to think that for nurses the strongest possible form of industrial action is a public declaration that we renounce it."

For those who still have the scars to show I like to think that the care and treatment they received was of the highest standard and quality that we were able to give.🗣

Community nursing 1973 and after

" *When working in the community it was essential to be in possession of local knowledge. This, combined with good intuition, helped to avoid potentially risky situations."*

District Nurse

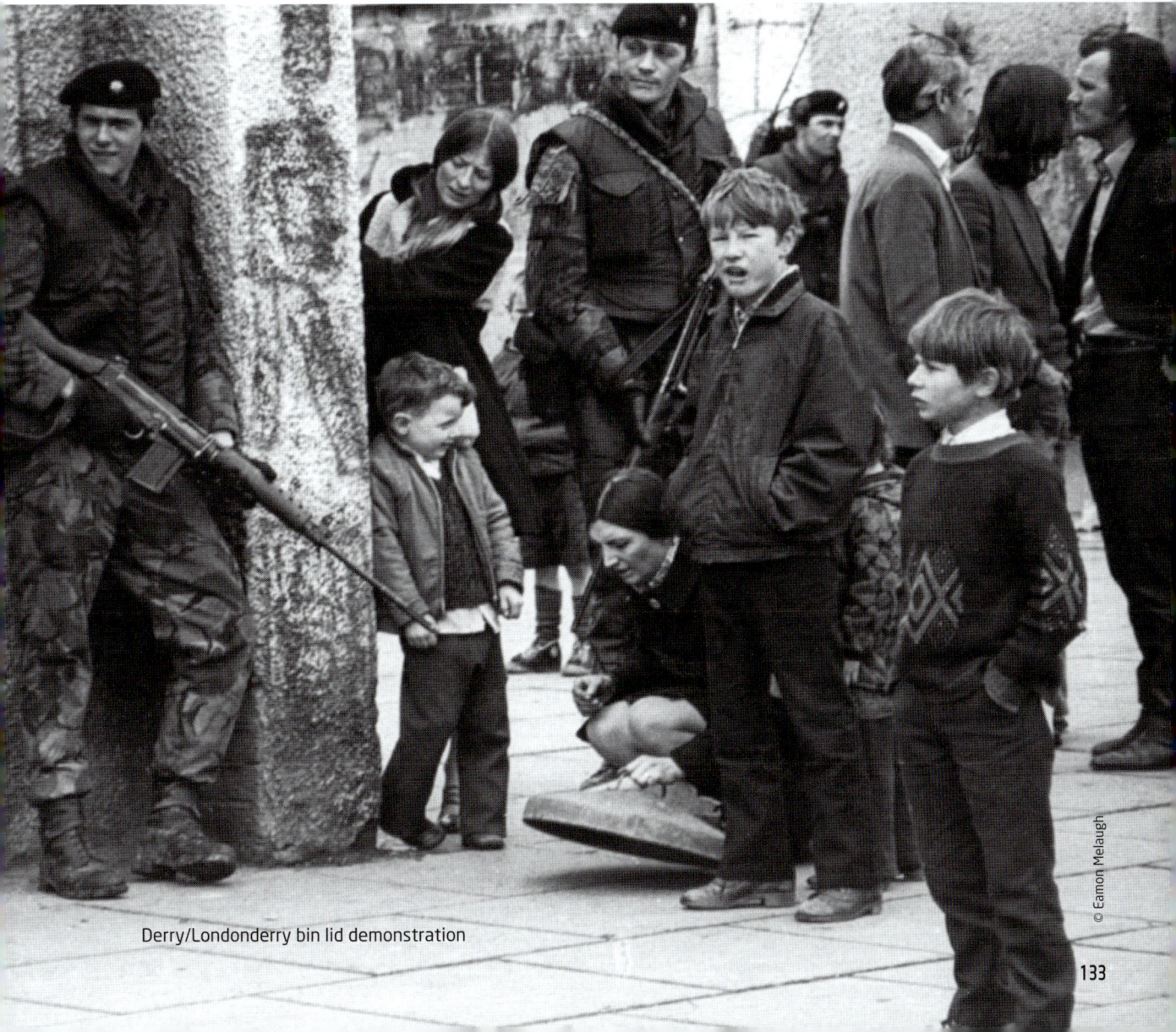

Derry/Londonderry bin lid demonstration

© Eamon Melaugh

133

"Unlike the Royal Victoria Hospital, which understandably attracted attention for its success in surgery and medicine treating casualties of the Troubles, community nursing remained, as Cinderellas do, in the background. Yet the diabetics received their insulin, the elderly had their dressings done and babies were weighed at clinic. Community nursing went on then as it does today."[1]

When the *Troubles erupted in 1969 responsibility for community nursing lay with city and county health authorities. In 1973, following a major restructuring of public services, four Health and Social Services Boards were established to commission and administer services to their assigned population. Community nurse management moved into newly created Units of Management which were commissioned to deliver health and social services. These subsequently had a number of managerial changes including the establishment of trusts. The commissioning board structure remained in place until 2009.*

"The civil unrest that was convulsing Northern Ireland actually had minimal impact on the implementation of the board scheme. Public health professionals carried out their duties despite severe travel disruption caused by street violence and bombings."[2]

Throughout the Troubles, community nurses worked across the province. Whilst the delivery of nursing services was relatively peaceful in many parts, delivering care and travelling around other areas could prove very demanding.

Some areas, because of the unpredictability of sporadic violence, were particularly challenging. This included North and West Belfast, the Bogside and Creggan in Derry/Londonderry, housing estates that by reputation had strong paramilitary association and border areas such as South Armagh and South Fermanagh.

As these stories were gathered, nurses who worked in some of these areas commented how stigmatised they felt because they had chosen to work in these localities. Some felt labelled as being sympathetic to the loyalties of the local community in which they worked while others felt colleagues elsewhere considered them not to be a "good" nurse as no sane person would willingly choose to work in the midst of such civil unrest.

"We were all targeted... parents of students would ring me before their placement... we looked after them well – both religions... students loved their placement" commented a community nurse working in an area of unrest, echoing sentiments expressed by other community nurses working in such locations.

Communities frequently identified themselves by painting kerbstones red, white and blue in Loyalist areas or green, white and orange in Republican areas. The gable murals of both communities, now tourist attractions, were a signal of

---

[1]All in a Day's work (1984) Nursing Times. December 5.

[2]Four Decades of Public Health – Northern Ireland's Health Boards 1973-2009. Public Health Agency, Belfast.

the local affiliation. All nurses were part of Northern Irish society and could be immediately identified by patients and clients as Protestant or Catholic – "one of us" or "one of them". Subtle cues, such as their name, certain pronunciations, and knowledge of local schools and churches could reveal a person's background.[3] Community nurses were fully aware of these nuances and adopted a non-partisan approach. They learnt to keep their focus on the task in hand rather than their surroundings. Many reported how families would advise them to avoid the area when trouble was expected.

Families associated with the security forces liked to know who was visiting and often requested no students. Mostly nurses were welcomed by all households and because they were providing care they did not feel directly threatened. Health was, in the main, a neutral topic.

Working with families under threat

❝I worked as a health visitor in an area that had a large number of police and security forces. These families were under severe and sustained threat from the IRA. We never took any students to visit or gave anyone access to these families. On their child health records the father's occupation was recorded as civil servant or similar as it was too dangerous to identify them as security or police.

---

[3]Mason C (1991) Working in a divided community. Nursing Standard. 6, 11.

As well as the stress that the fathers were under, mothers carried a huge burden in protecting their families. No work clothes could be hung on the washing line. All had to be dried inside without the benefit of tumble dryers or central heating in the early days. Clothes were ironed after children had gone to bed; there could be no sign which led to suspicion. Uniforms were kept in locked wardrobes.

Children were told fathers did office jobs and had to be away at times on business. The reality was that many were working in extremely dangerous situations with the very real threat of death. There was also the problem of the security of legally held weapons. It was difficult for mothers to continue as normal.

Many of them had little family support in Belfast with relatives living far away and often reluctant to travel. As is the way with families, each had their own individual problems, to a greater or lesser extent.

I recall visiting one family with a severely disabled child with complex needs. The little boy cried in a high-pitched tone most of the time. I knew the strain on the family was immense. They had little family support and the father was away from home for long periods, especially when tensions were high in the community.

I visited frequently. One day I called at about 10am. The mother and I were in the living room with the little boy when the front door opened and I heard someone run up stairs. It was the husband and the mother went to get his supper as he was home from night duty. She had just rejoined me when there was a crash and the back door flew open. She ran into the kitchen to find the dinner thrown against the window.

Her husband ran down the garden, fell on his knees and started to howl with his head in his arms. I will never forget the sight of that tiny mother trying to comfort her large husband who was so clearly in great distress. The noise upset the little boy who started to cry in a very agitated manner. I called the GP and asked for an urgent visit and asked one of my colleagues to get in touch with a friend of the family to take the boy.

I stayed until the GP left and tried to settle the family down as best I could. It transpired that the husband had seen some colleagues of his killed.

A few years later the family moved away. I often wondered what became of them.**"**

Dressing continues

"As a nursing student on a community placement I was kneeling down doing an elderly lady's leg ulcer dressings (liquid paraffin wraps!) at a wee kitchen house in North Belfast. This was during a riot with bin lids banging and shots flying.

Next thing, two gunmen burst through the rear of the house from the entry, raced through the room and out the front door. Dressing continues! We just looked at one another and I realised how resilient these elderly residents were despite the daily trauma of paramilitary activity.**"**

Community nursing in Portadown

"I worked as a district nurse and midwife in Portadown from 1968-1975. When the riots started in the town there was absolute turmoil. Cars were being taken from their drivers and overturned, burned and smashed. But I have to say I never had a problem, and was treated with the utmost respect, and never was hindered from doing my work.

I was treated with courtesy from both sides of the community. It was a great team of community nurses to work with and it didn't make any difference what religion we were.**"**

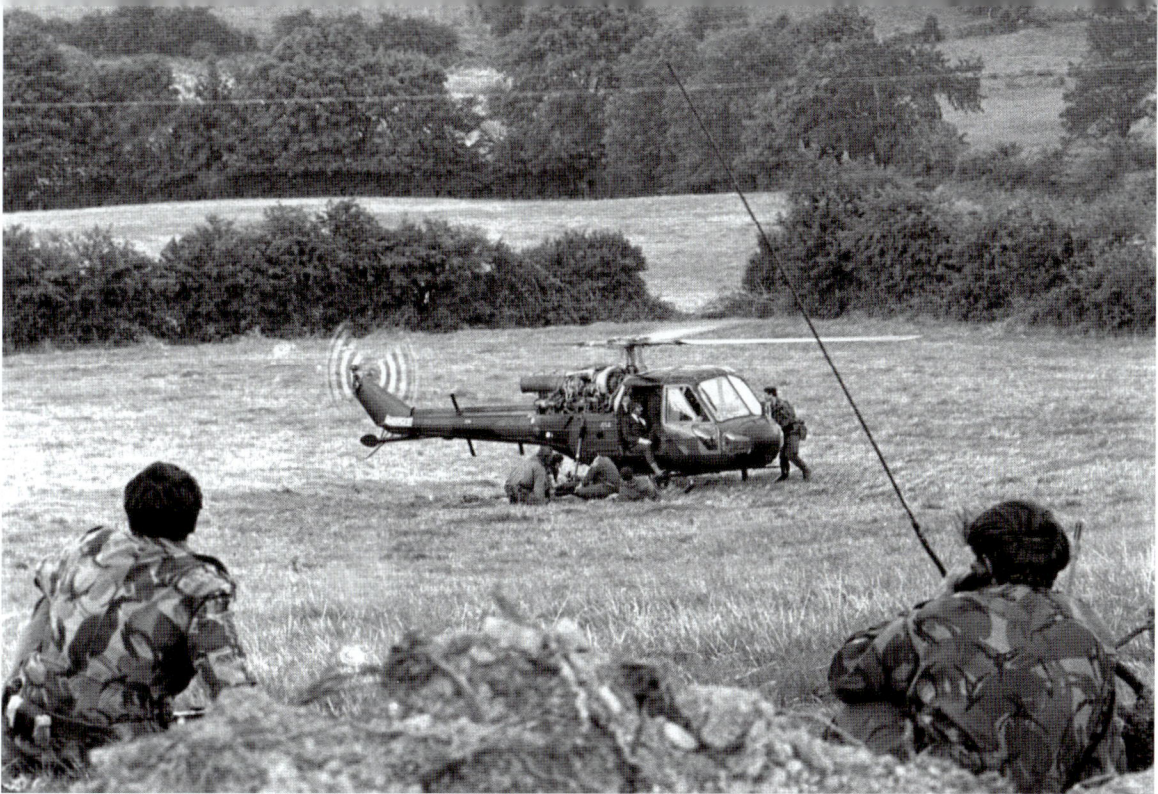

Crossmaglen, army helicopter

Mistaken identity

"Travelling alone to a patient's home one morning I observed a low-flying helicopter with its doors open at close range. I stopped my car.

As the helicopter flew over, a rope was lowered to the road. It was difficult to see or hear due to the noise and dust of the landing helicopter. Two soldiers emerged down the rope and ran towards my car.

One soldier pointed his gun at me while the second soldier walked towards me, ordering me from my car. I felt shocked and vulnerable. The soldier was clearly nervous, his hands shaking, as he shouted commands at me. Pinned against the door of the car, with my hands upright, the soldier demanded identification, which I produced promptly. I knew my life was in danger as I stood inches from the barrel of his gun. Informing him

I was a community nurse, I spoke calmly, knowing the situation could change at any minute. I was shaking in my shoes.

His companion searched my car. I looked at the soldier as he circled around and he reminded me of my young son. I thought of my family, and wondered if this was the place I was going to die.

After I answered his questions, the soldier radioed my identification in code, while I remained at gunpoint, terrified. Consulting with his colleague, the pair slowly lowered their guns and the aggressive mood changed. One soldier informed me that my car had been mistaken for a similar vehicle, which was involved in a bank raid that morning. They handed me back my identification and I was told to proceed. Without speaking, both soldiers ran to their waiting helicopter. Trembling I got into my car and drove to my patient's home.

Returning later to the medical centre I informed my nurse manager. Though emotionally distressed, I remained on duty. No counselling or psychological services were available.

The police called to see my husband and offered an apology for the distress caused. They added that procedures would be reviewed to ensure such a mistake would not happen again. Within days I received a written apology with a bouquet of flowers. It was good to be alive to smell the flowers! Talking with colleagues later they joked that it was like a scene from a James Bond movie. Over four decades, I nursed many people who experienced great tragedy and loss. Despite the turmoil and disruption, patients were always my first concern. Striving to maintain high standards of nursing care, I treated each one as an individual, always respecting their tradition and their dignity.**"**

Growing up with the Troubles

"Children growing up in the unstable environment of the 1970s and 1980s never failed to amaze me with their stoic resilience. They played with their peers and mock guns round the security barriers and at the soldiers' feet at times – sometimes cheeky and sometimes friendly with them.

I have seen a little girl totally absorbed, sweeping the footpath outside her house with her mother's broom when a security alert was in progress not half a block away. Scars might, and did, show up in later life, but that was still in the future.

On one homeward journey our cars were held up by a bomb scare at a nearby high-rise block of flats. Unconcerned children continued to play hide and seek and a game of 'tig' round the building while the security search continued. Incidents like these just became the norm for both children and commuters alike.

For my part, working in a conflict area was challenging but never dull – frustrating at times but also very rewarding.**"**

On nobody's side

"Many estate families had no involvement at all in 'irregular' activities. Indeed many mothers tried to keep their young people out of it, not an easy task with young adolescents who relished the excitement of a riot.

When their menfolk were 'lifted' or imprisoned or hiding over the border, mothers still had to put food on the table and many resented having to cope single-handedly. Until money started to flow in from abroad, particularly the USA, unpaid bills were a way of life.

Once on a visit to a family home where the husband had just been interrogated for suspected involvement in paramilitary activities, which he was denying emphatically to me, his wife retorted: 'He's in it up to his neck, nurse,' and then, to him: 'Stop lying to her – she's a nurse and she's on nobody's side.'

This is indeed how a nurse should be, but it must be recognised that none of us comes baggage-free. Being the recipient of certain inside confidential information, as we sometimes inadvertently were, could at times lead to moral, ethical or legal dilemmas for us. We had little in the way of guidance or counselling from management on coping with delicate issues, trying to maintain client relationships while at the same time staying within the law."

The mobile coronary care unit

In 1965 Professor Pantridge, Cardiology Consultant at the Royal Victoria Hospital, had developed the world's first portable defibrillator, which had been installed into an ambulance. This mobile coronary care unit was based in the coronary care wards in the Royal and staff were specially trained to go out on the cardiac ambulance, which was on call 24 hours a day to treat patients in the community. The following stories are from nurses who travelled with this unit.

Tin helmets

"I worked as a part-time staff nurse on the cardiac unit (wards 5 and 6) at RVH at the end of 1969 and the start of the Troubles. Part of my role was to ride the cardiac ambulance on emergency calls. This ambulance was normally staffed with a registrar, a staff nurse and a medical student along with a hospital driver.

During these years roads were often blocked off and traffic disrupted. Those in the ambulance had to wear special headgear to protect them from any attack. This headgear

was similar to the round tin helmets used by street wardens in World War Two – only these were white with a red cross on the front.

One night at about 11.30pm the cardiac ambulance was called out to a lady living on a housing estate in West Belfast who was complaining of severe chest pain. On our way to the given address we were stopped by men wearing black clothes, balaclavas and carrying rifles. The doctor explained we were going to an emergency call. One of the men ordered us to turn back stating that no one was allowed past them. The doctor pointed out that we were an emergency team and it was of the utmost importance that we get to the patient quickly. The men then opened our ambulance back doors to see the occupants and ensure we were who we said we were. Eventually we were permitted to proceed but with one of the men riding on the running board of the ambulance.

When we arrived at the house we were not allowed to go in until the man confirmed with the occupants that we had been called to attend the lady. As we tried to enter the house the man attempted to come in with us but the doctor said we needed to see the patient privately and for the man to come in would be unethical as well as stressful for the lady concerned. The man reluctantly agreed to stand outside the front door but was not happy at having to do so.

When the doctor decided we should take the patient with us to hospital for observation the man said this was not allowed! He was made aware that he would be responsible for anything which might happen to the patient and that we had a duty of care to bring her to hospital. We were allowed to proceed but again the man accompanied us on the running board of the ambulance until he reached the main road when he at last dismounted.

This was a very scary time but because it was our job we did not really think about the danger we were faced with until we were back in the safety of our beloved RVH.

Incidentally, the patient was diagnosed with severe angina and went on to make a good recovery. **"**

The living and the dead

"When I worked as a staff nurse and junior sister on the coronary care and cardiology ward at the Royal Victoria Hospital Belfast, I was part of the cardiac ambulance team. Late one Sunday morning, usually a quiet time, the bright-red emergency phone rang to request the cardiac ambulance.

On answering the phone I discovered that a local GP had been called to a house where a 28-year-old man had collapsed. The GP thought the man was dead but the family and neighbours who had gathered outside this house, on a housing estate, were both upset and angry. We said that we would come immediately.

The hospital switchboard bleeped the cardiac ambulance team members and we all ran to meet the ambulance in a staff car park nearby. We assembled the necessary equipment to deal with a collapse as we sped along a main road, before turning into the maze of streets and eventually arriving at the correct house.

A crowd of about 30 men, women and children had assembled on the pavement and road outside the house. We were met by the GP and family members. Some of them were shouting: 'Come on, hurry up, what kept you?' The team rushed upstairs following the GP into the patient's bedroom, carrying all the necessary equipment.

It was immediately evident that this young man had been dead for many hours. He had come in late on Saturday night having had a lot to drink and had lain down fully clothed on his bed. During the night he had vomited and inhaled his vomit, thus obstructing his airway, causing death.

Due to the extreme agitation of the family, the GP and the crowd outside the house, the team took the unusual decision to try to resuscitate this man although they knew he was dead. Resuscitation attempts including defibrillation continued for about five minutes before the Registrar announced that the patient was dead. The man's family were informed of his death and a local priest arrived to be with the family.

The team left the house to return to the hospital past an initially silent and then quietly angry and sullen crowd. A few people were saying: 'What use were you... you took so long?' In this situation we had been presented with a moral and ethical dilemma.

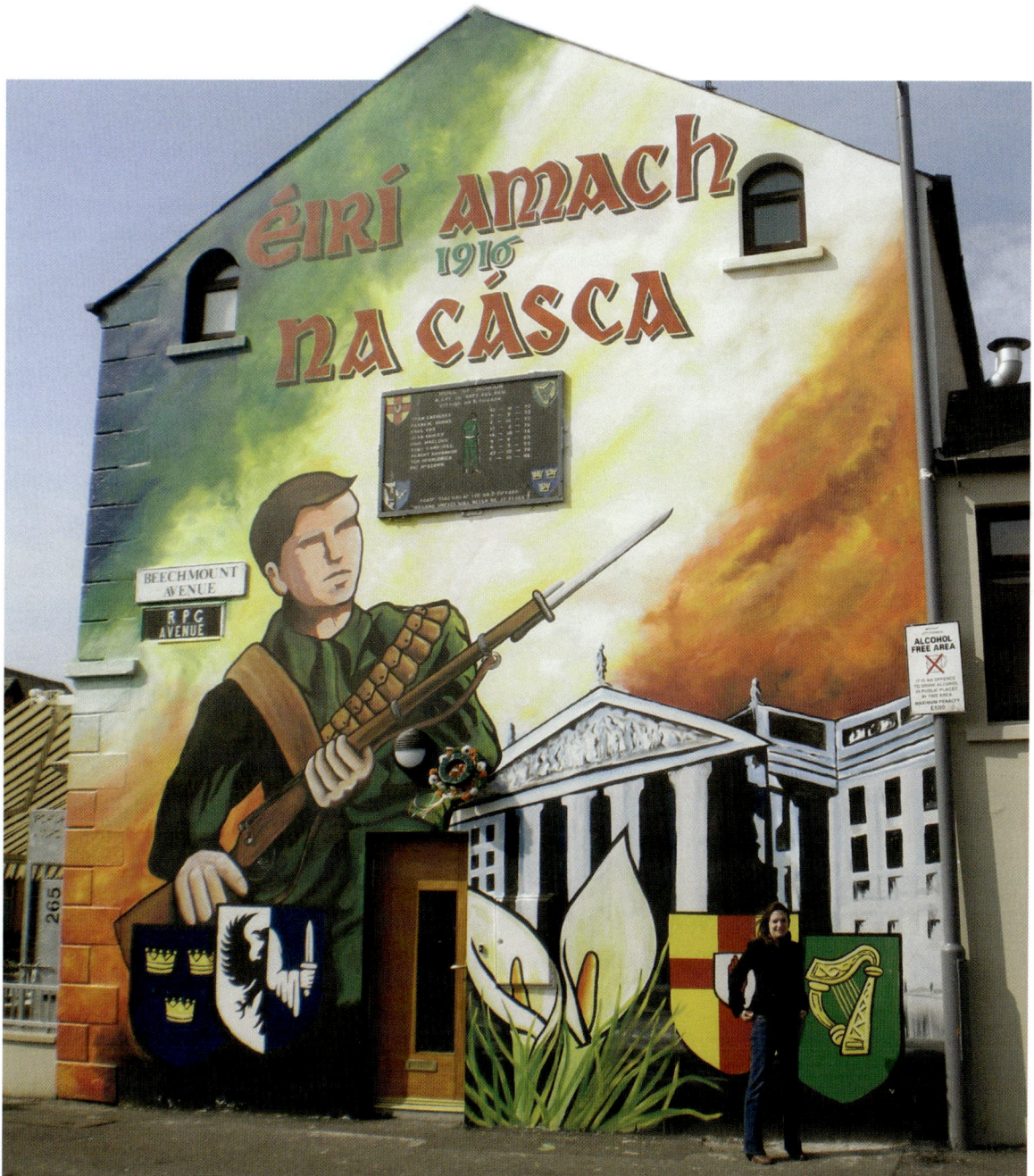

Republican Easter lily mural

When the GP telephoned he knew that his patient was dead but he was scared that the family and the crowd would be aggressive towards him as the patient was a leading paramilitary and very influential in the neighbourhood. So the cardiac ambulance team had to go through the motions of a resuscitation attempt to ensure the GP's current safety and future ability to practise in that area.

This 'utilitarian' approach to ethics ensured the greatest good for the greatest number and was undoubtedly the right thing to do in these difficult circumstances. 🙶

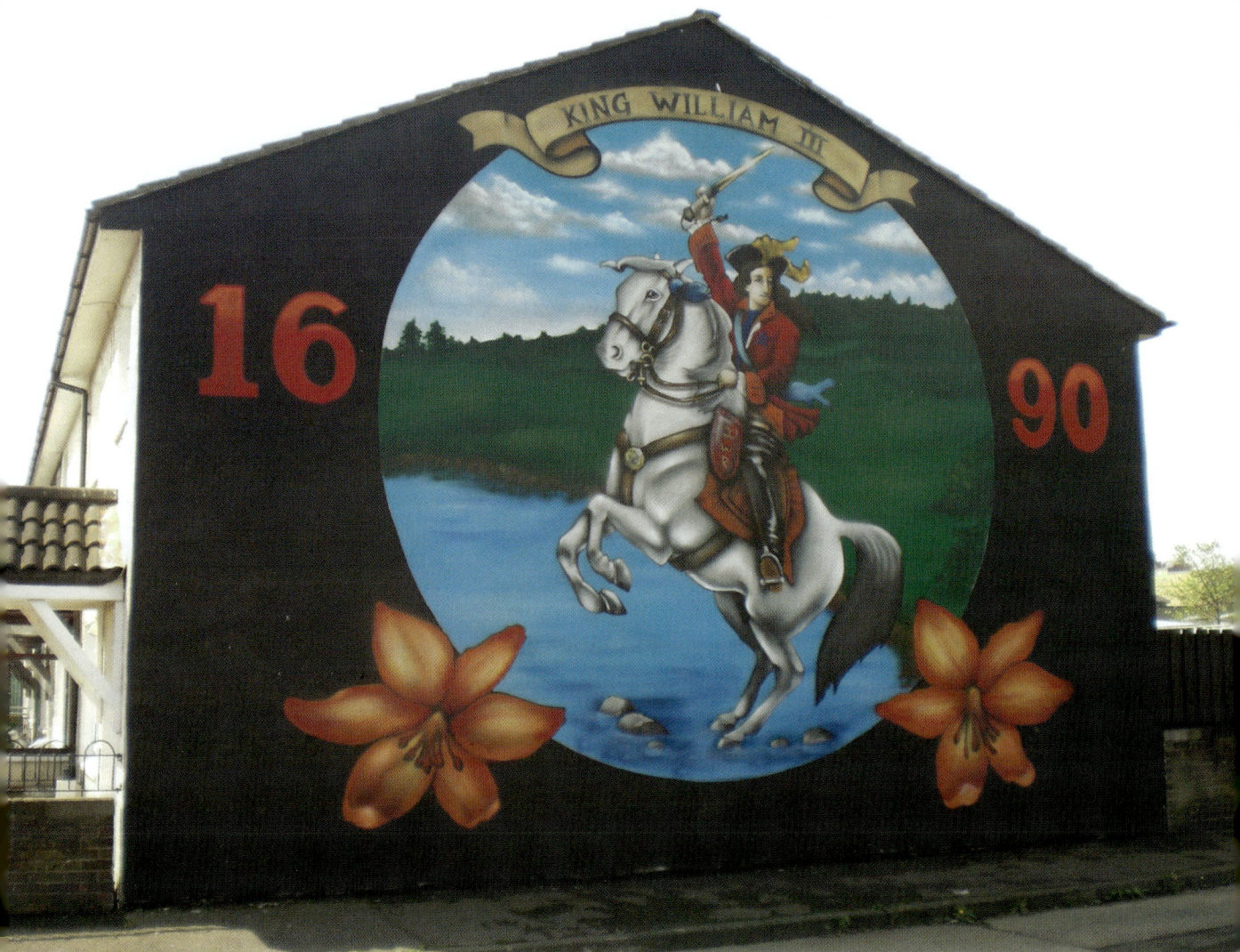

Loyalist King Billy mural

Night duty

"During my staffing years I worked on the cardiac ambulance during the Ulster Workers Council strike in May 1974. These were anxious and nervous days as we had to depend on the good will of those manning the barricades to make our way through parts of Belfast.

During the hunger strikes I again was working night duty on the cardiac ambulance and at that time there were many barricades on the streets making it hazardous getting to calls. Seeing children fill bottles with petrol, yards from where rounds of plastic bullets were being fired, will always remain in my memory. On one occasion bringing in a patient we arrived just minutes after shots had been fired at soldiers on duty at the ward entrance. We were so lucky not to have been caught up in it.

I feel privileged to have worked in the Royal during these years. We are part of history."

Major incidents 1980-1989

" *There were continual funerals; I remember the silence in the town. Nurses went to the funerals; many of the dead were their friends.*"

Casualty Sister

Enniskillen bomb, 1987

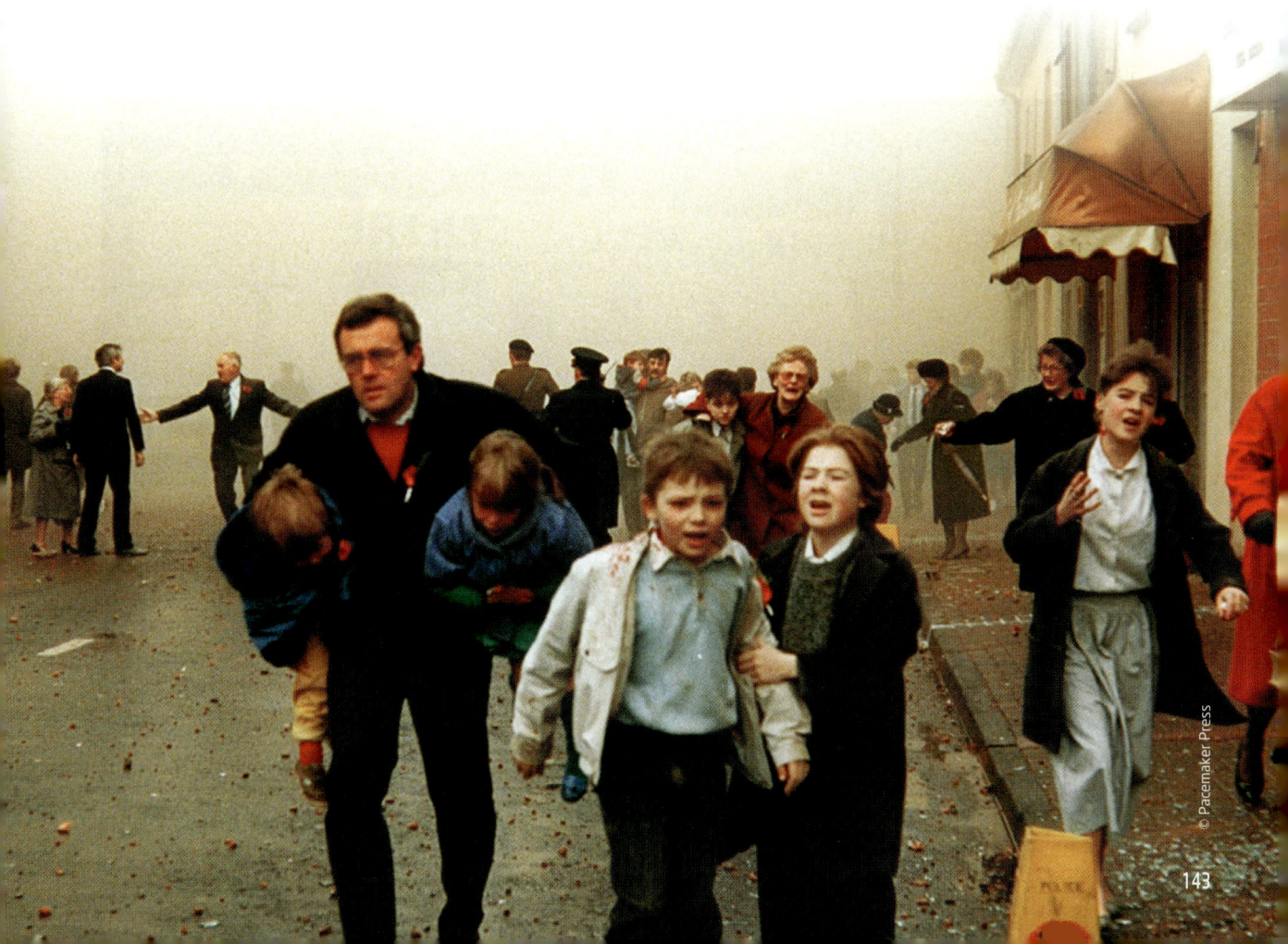

© Pacemaker Press

143

1980-1989
Deaths 853
Injured 9,554

Violence continued through the 1970s and into the 1980s. Patterns of violence changed and the number of indiscriminate bombings of towns and cities fell while paramilitary attacks became more focused on security personnel and their bases. Paramilitary sectarian attacks from both sides of the community were frequently carried out almost on a 'tit for tat' basis.

Many nurses who had worked in front line services throughout the 1970s remained in post and continued to support new intakes of students.

Droppin' Well Bomb, Ballykelly, 6 December 1982

A bomb killed 17 people in the Droppin' Well Disco and Bar in Ballykelly, County Derry/Londonderry. More than 30 people were injured. Injuries were the result of fallen masonry as the bomb caused the roof to collapse.

"In 1982 I was closely involved in the aftermath of the bomb at the Droppin' Well Disco at Ballykelly, a village where the Shackleton army barracks was based.

Messages were relayed over the radio and television for all available staff to come into the hospital to help with the bomb victims.

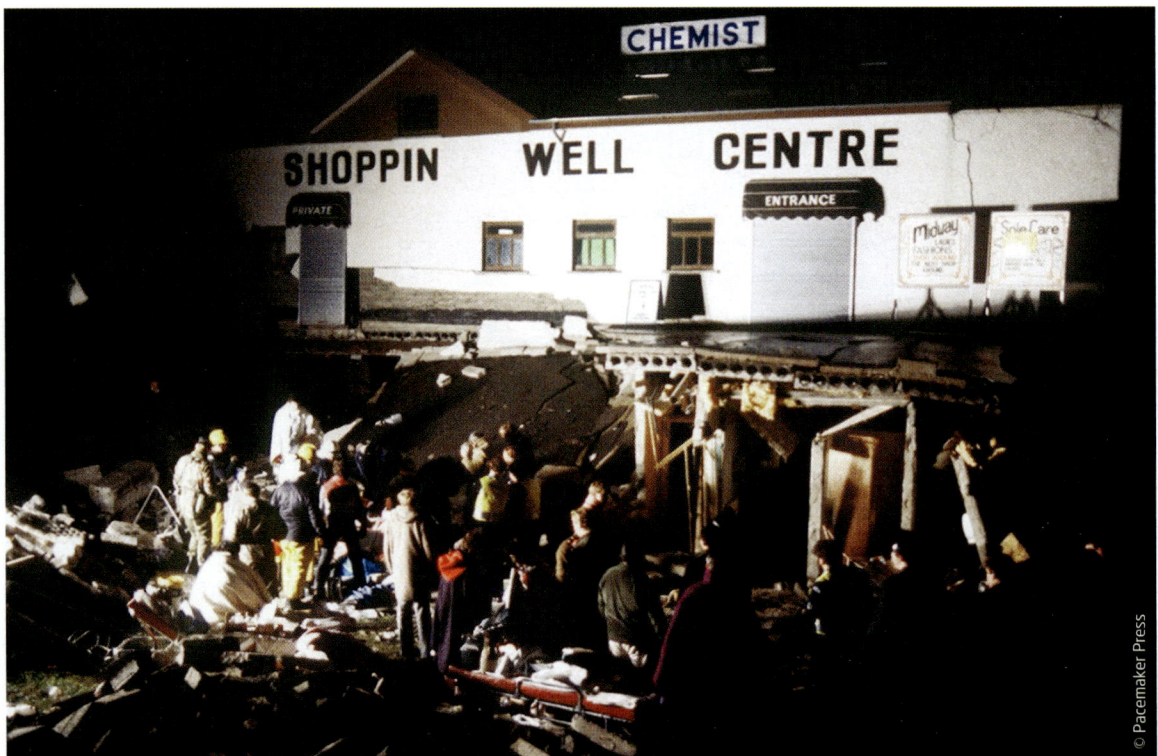

Ballykelly Droppin' Well Disco bombing, 1982

© Pacemaker Press

I was on day duty, and was sister in charge of A&E theatre. The sight that met me as I entered the ground corridor of the hospital was beds and trolleys lined up with casualties suffering with various injuries. The consultant in charge, Mr Bennett, was assessing the casualties, directing some to theatres. Any that could be treated or needed urgent resuscitation were kept in casualty and A&E theatre.

A few hours later we were advised that there was still at least one soldier trapped under rubble. A team consisting of myself, a staff nurse, an orthopaedic consultant, Mr Gavin Price, and an anaesthetist, Dick McErlean, were asked to go out to the bomb scene with the intention of, if necessary, amputating the soldier's trapped legs.

Arriving at the site it was an eerie scene. Being now around 1am, it was cold and dark and the only light was coming from arc lights rigged by the firemen who were still battling to release the casualty. He was trapped under masonry – huge concrete boulders which looked immovable. We crawled in to reach the patient, gave him morphine and kept him as warm as we could while reassuring him that he would be freed as soon as possible.

The firemen were magnificent using heavy lifting machinery and cutting equipment. Eventually, after about four hours, we had him on a stretcher in the ambulance and transferred safely to the hospital with his limbs intact.

We had come prepared for any eventuality, including amputation if necessary, but we were very glad that we did not have to carry out any surgery on site because of the dust and dirt. Nevertheless we had a sense of great achievement having saved his life on that occasion. He, like others, was repatriated to England.

On that night there were 27 people injured needing hospital treatment. Thankfully they survived and went home, though probably never to be the same again. Seventeen others were not so lucky. Eleven soldiers of the Cheshire regiment and six civilians were killed, one of whom was the owner's daughter. Three of the dead were teenagers. They were all out celebrating Christmas.

I became involved in politics in 1985 and was asked to be part of a group 'We too have suffered'. I met the mother of one of the young girls killed at Ballykelly and other parents who had lost loved ones in the Troubles as well as others whose lives were also shattered.**"**

Enniskillen Poppy Day Bomb, 8 November 1987

Eleven people were killed and 63 injured, some seriously when an IRA bomb exploded at the town's war memorial during the annual Remembrance Sunday ceremony.

"That Sunday many people gathered in Enniskillen to attend the Remembrance Service held at 11am at the cenotaph. But a peaceful Sunday morning became the scene of devastating carnage when, at 10.45am, a 30lb IRA bomb exploded in a disused building just behind where many elderly folk and local families stood waiting for the service to commence.

I was off-duty from my role as Assistant Director of Nursing at the Erne Hospital. My telephone rang alerting me to the major tragedy unfolding. I immediately returned to the hospital to join colleagues providing nursing care and comfort for the injured as the casualties poured in.

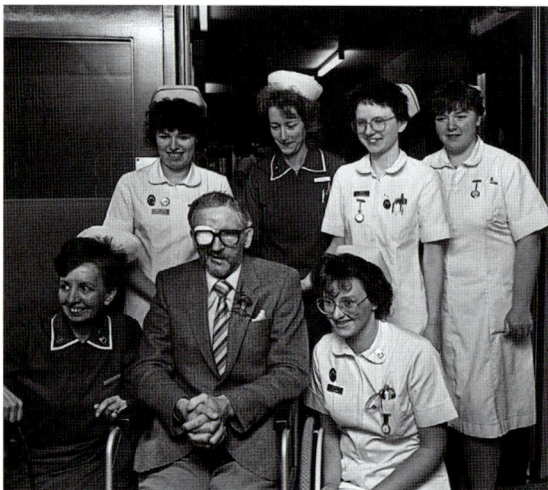

© Pacemaker Press

Enniskillen bomb, 1987 - survivor with nurses

Most of the nurses in the Erne Hospital, which has 248 beds, had experience of caring for victims of violence, but this was very different. Many of the staff knew those who had been killed or injured. Some of the more seriously hurt were stabilised and transferred to other hospitals by helicopter.

As the hospital was a short distance from the cenotaph, relatives were arriving before the injured. Because of the major injuries, dust and state of shock, it was very difficult to identify the casualties.

There was a temporary mortuary set up and I can remember a very senior nursing colleague contacting me and asking how she could help. She kindly went to the mortuary and communicated essential accurate details to me. It was very stressful having to tell relatives that a loved one had been killed or very seriously injured.

Many of the dead had a close connection with the hospital. One was a retired ambulance driver and his wife had been a nurse in the treatment room of the adjoining health centre. Another victim was a retired nursing sister and one was a lovely student nurse in training. An elderly gentleman who visited the hospital weekly and brought gifts to the patients at Christmas was also killed.

Those who were left to grieve were in deep shock and that was true of the whole town, in fact the whole county. Being a close-knit community, people were numbed by what had occurred. That was even more true of the hospital staff trying

Survivors greet the royal couple

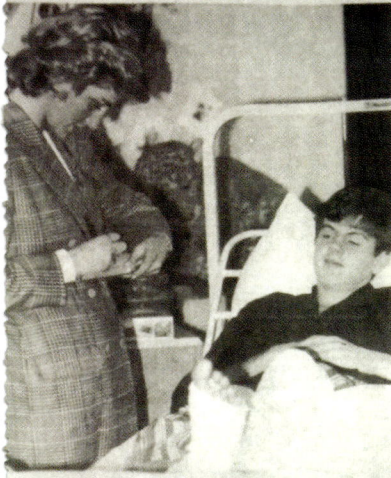

With a victim: The Princess of Wales gives her autograph to Nathan Chambers, aged 15.

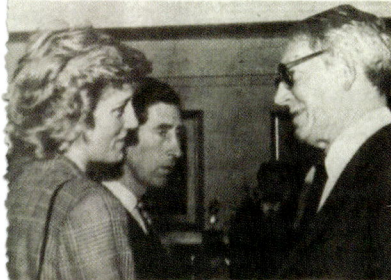

With the bereaved: The royal couple meet Mr Gordon Wilson, who lost his daughter Marie.

A royal visit – Princeess Diana and Prince Charles.
The Times 1987

to fulfil their medical and nursing duties while dealing with their own sense of an overwhelming bereavement and shock.

Some young children who were injured have fully recovered and have gone on to pursue successful careers. Others who were hurt sadly have not made a full recovery and still require surgery.

Later the International Rotary Club gave money to provide a new chaplain's and relatives' room and furnished it beautifully. The nursing staff and chaplains met regularly for discussions and openly expressed their feelings.

Many people called at the hospital to thank the staff and to encourage them. One lady of 80 years sent a cheque for £100 for the staff. We arranged a special afternoon tea for staff and held it outside as the weather was fine. This treat was enjoyed by all grades of staff. Also a lovely bouquet of flowers arrived for the staff from colleagues at the Royal Victoria Hospital.

Prince Charles and Princess Diana visited the hospital and this was a tremendous boost to both staff and patient morale. However it will take many, many years before that sense of loss and grief entirely disappears. **"**

"Go to our house and switch off the oven - please"

A sister recalls...

"The local Erne Hospital had opened in 1964. It was a 248-bed unit with 38 surgical beds. It had four high-dependency beds and one intensive care bed.

The accident and emergency unit had been extended to provide six additional cubicles fitted with oxygen and suction. An operating theatre was adjacent to the unit. We were fortunate to have a large physiotherapy department fitted with emergency equipment next to A&E as this allowed for an overflow of patients and their relatives during major incidents.

The peace of Enniskillen was first disturbed by bombing incidents in 1970 and continued until the Ceasefire. On Remembrance Sunday 1987 I was at home and heard the bomb blast at the cenotaph. I saw smoke and immediately phoned the hospital switchboard, informed them of the bomb and instructed the staff nurse on duty to implement the major disaster plan. We had an emergency cupboard with prepared notes and I gave her the details then dashed to the hospital. Staffing that day was a staff nurse and plaster orderly.

The place was full of distressed relatives looking for their loved ones and waiting for news. Many were my friends. The full horror soon hit, the large number of killed and injured. I knew many of them. Mrs Quentin, a nurse in the army; Jessie, a nurse who had just retired and had said: 'I want to enjoy retirement'; the chemist and his wife... all friends of ours. The deaths and injuries were caused by falling masonry.

We had to be strong and carry on. Gordon Wilson asked me: 'Where's Marie... find Marie. I'm alright.' Marie was his daughter and a student nurse. I didn't know she was one of the first admitted and was in theatre.

Those that needed looking after were in the consulting rooms but we couldn't keep them in there... It was organised chaos, but there was no panic. Everyone was in deep shock. So many asked for phone calls to be made to get someone to turn their ovens off... but it was impossible to meet these requests.

Staff seemed to just appear. Many of my nursing colleagues knew patients that were injured and killed, all we could do was to comfort and support one another. So many other organisations helped that day, the clergy, police and army. Helicopters were used to transfer patients out to other hospitals.

Our disaster plan worked well. We were congratulated on our notes. We all got together in the tearoom afterwards; it took until 8pm to clear up and clean and check all the equipment. A few stayed on and we were relieved we coped as well as we did.

Afterwards there were continual funerals; I remember the silence in the town. Nurses went to the funerals; many of the dead were their friends.

Do you know my mother?
I remember one occasion while working at the A&E department of the Erne Hospital. Soldiers were brought in wounded. They had been celebrating a 21st birthday when a bomb went off. One died in casualty. Another young soldier I was looking after asked me: 'Do you know my mum? She has the same badge as you. Can you ring my mum and tell her I'm okay?' He survived. It was great that I could tell her he was going to be all right. "

Milltown Cemetery Attack, 16 March 1988

Mourners were attacked by a single gunman while attending the funerals of paramilitary volunteers. Three people were killed and more than 50 injured. The event was captured by television cameras.

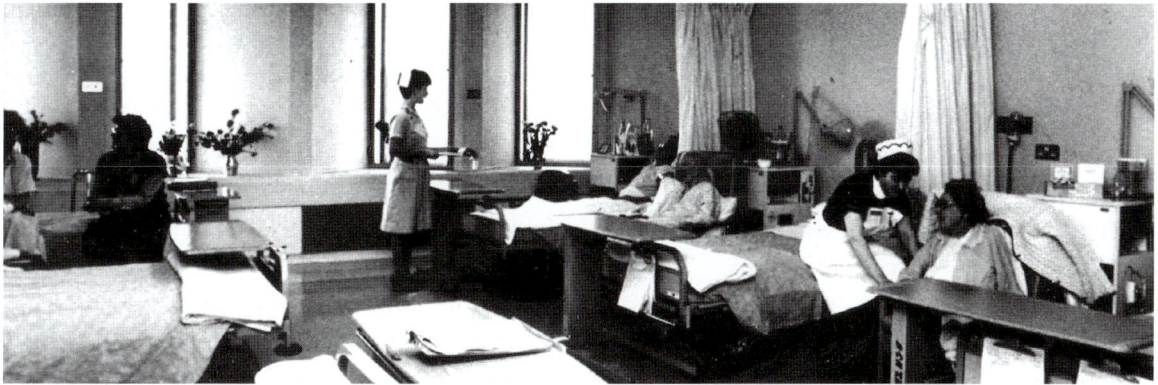

Belfast City Hospital, 1980s

Bullets on the floor

A staff nurse at Belfast City Hospital A&E remembers...

"An incident which is very clear in my mind is the attack in Milltown Cemetery. I was in the canteen having lunch when the phone rang asking for A&E staff to return to the department.

I was informed that there had been a number of casualties with blast and gunshot injuries brought in to hospital. I took up my position in the trauma room, and suddenly the police arrived with this big man with long dark hair, a beard and wearing a black boiler suit.

At first I thought he was a member of the special patrol group, a branch of the RUC, but soon realised he wasn't when the police started to question him as to where the other grenades were. I think I turned white as the police told me what had happened, and I was wondering if this man had more grenades on his person and whether he might try to explode one of them.

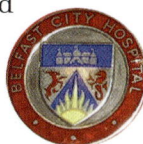

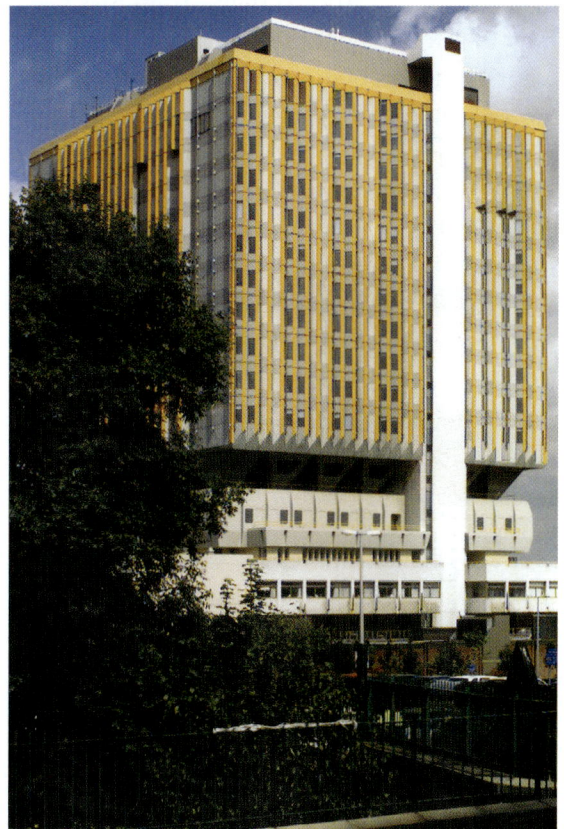

Belfast City Hospital, new tower block

I also remember when I was trying to take his clothing off – we always had to do this carefully and individually bag each item for forensic examination – a number of bullets fell onto the floor.**"**

Red alert

I started nursing in 1987 in the Royal Victoria Hospital alongside 53 other girls. My first real memory is of the Milltown Cemetery shooting, which was our first 'red alert'.

Even though we were still students in college we were on standby and expected to help when called upon to do so. This event showed me for the first time just how much a part of the Royal I was, and what high expectations were placed on me as a nurse.

I had never even worn my uniform at this time but the nurse tutor Ms McEvoy made it very clear that we were all expected to help in whatever role we were called up for. The fear of letting her down was probably greater than actually having to nurse the wounded. In the end we were not needed for this red alert but it was a huge lesson for all of us about what exactly we had signed up for from day one.**

Ballygawley Bus Bombing, 20 August 1988

A bomb attack on a bus carrying army personnel killed eight soldiers and injured 28.

I was working in Omagh Hospital on the night of the Ballygawley bomb. A staff nurse and I were on ward 7. It was a busy night and we had just settled down to paperwork and a cup of tea, when the night sister came round.

With panic in her voice she said to go to casualty immediately as we were needed for an emergency. My colleague suggested that I go as I had just returned from Saudi Arabia where I worked in trauma and fractures for two years.

I raced down to casualty thinking that I wouldn't know where anything was kept as I hadn't worked there before. It was utter mayhem. Lots of people in a small area and staff I didn't know. I just went to a trolley and one lad lay with his head partially covered in bandages.

He couldn't see me, but asked my name. I said: 'My name is Mary,' and held his hand. I don't remember his name but he just kept saying: 'Tell my mum I'm okay. Tell her I will be okay, tell her I'm okay.'

The consultant asked me to undress his wounds and half his face wasn't there – a sight I will never forget. I held his hand for what seemed like ages until he was transferred to a Belfast hospital. I thought he looked about 18 years old, and he just wanted his mum. I never found out what happened to him.**

Intensive care nursing through the 1980s

I was appointed Senior Sister in the respiratory and intensive care unit in 1981. This was in the middle of the Troubles and dealing with the aftermath of bombings and shootings was at times a daily occurrence. However we just got on with it and, in a strange way, it became a way of life.

We all supported each other, worked well together as a team and learnt so much as a result of dealing with victims and their families.

The unit was heavily secured. In the early days the British army guarded the unit and then in the mid-1980s the RUC provided regular security for all of us, victims and perpetrators alike.

Security intensified after a sniper was seen one evening on the roof of the Royal Maternity Hospital and an RUC officer was shot dead in the unit. From then on we were kept safe behind bulletproof glass and secure doors. We came to know the security guards and indeed a number of the nurses met their future husbands from among the guards.

I remember so many of the terrorists who ended up in the unit, even some who are now in government in Northern Ireland. It was usually their relatives who required more effort in managing than the actual patients. Dr Gray's humour over these years was greatly appreciated and his quiet and unassuming leadership was key to the unit being a very happy and harmonious place to work. We all appreciated that so much.

I remember a well-known senior Loyalist being admitted one night following a fight in Belfast. He had to go to theatre to have a mid sternotomy and repair of his diaphragm. An Indian surgical registrar took him to theatre and had to cut through a full chest-sized tattoo of King Billy on his horse.

On reviewing the patient the next morning, Dr Gray said to me: 'Mr Kumar has made a good job of King Billy – the tattoo has made it easier to make sure he was sewn up correctly!'

I remember the hunger strikers who had multiple guards around them at all times and this made nursing so much more difficult. The pressure was always there. We didn't know what might happen next and we had to always be ready for any emergency.

The Remembrance Sunday in Enniskillen when the bomb went off was particularly sad. A nursing officer came to tell me that one of our student nurses, Marie Wilson, had been caught up in the tragedy. I remember Marie attending the Royal choir the previous Tuesday evening, and being stunned that she was now a victim of the bomb blast. We admitted a number of the victims from Enniskillen that evening.

On another occasion I remember being annoyed that 'relatives' had deceived us into believing that they were related to a 14-year-old boy from Londonderry who had been hit by a plastic bullet. Two ladies arrived at the door of the unit shortly before he died and they told me they were his aunts and wanted in to see him. I let them in and then suddenly noticed them taking out a large camera, taking a photograph and then running out of the unit. I ran with a colleague after them but to no avail.

To my shock, the photograph appeared on the local news that evening. By this stage, the young boy was dead.

Clinitron therapy

The trauma we witnessed often meant we were dealing with injuries that hadn't been seen before in Northern Ireland, or indeed in the UK. I remember the day we had a call from Daisy Hill Hospital in Newry about a man who was a victim of a bomb under his car seat, triggered when he switched on the ignition. He had lost his buttocks and lower aspects of both thighs. I remember thinking: How on earth would we manage to nurse someone on a bed with such injuries?'

The previous month one of my colleagues and I had been at a conference in London and we had seen a new therapy bed called the Clinitron bed. It was a bed or tank filled with very fine silicon beads that moved gently to reduce the pressure on the skin and allowed wound exudate to drain cleanly away. I immediately thought that this bed might assist this patient, so I rang the company and asked them to get a bed to us for the next day.

They politely told me that this wouldn't be possible, but that they might be able to get it to us the following week. I told them that if they wanted to do business with us, they needed to get the bed on the Liverpool boat that night and get it to the unit for the following day. And guess what, they delivered!

That was the beginning of an important partnership and the company set up business in Northern Ireland the following year, and are still here. I remember travelling with two of the consultants to the World Intensive Care Conference in Kyoto, Japan in 1989 to deliver a paper on the benefits of Clinitron therapy for bomb blast victims.

I also remember a lovely girl, Karen, being admitted one Saturday night after being hit by a bullet at close range in her neck. She had been singing at a gospel meeting in East Belfast that evening and after the event, a gunman came up to her in her boyfriend's car and shot her. She was paralysed immediately. Despite her tragic story she was an amazing person. She lived for another three weeks and I was with her when she died.

Karen made a huge impact on all the staff, especially the nurses. She was always smiling and spoke of her hope and forgiveness for the gunman. Her family were equally brave. Her sister-in-law had a baby just before Karen died. I remember the family asking me to tell her the news. I'm not sure if Karen heard me, but her story touched us all.

The constant pressure

The Monday after the Musgrave Park bomb went off in the military wing, I was walking through the nurses' station when the phone rang. I answered and was told that the IRA had just phoned the switchboard to advise that they had planted a bomb in the unit. We had admitted some of the injured soldiers over the weekend and the IRA viewed us as a target.

One of the consultants who was doing a ward round at the time said he wasn't going to evacuate the ward. If we had done so, it was likely that some of the very unstable and critically ill patients could have died in the decant. The army came in and did a search of the unit and basement below us. While nothing was found, it was yet another example of the pressure staff lived under each day.

I always remember my father warning me to check under my car every evening when I went off the unit to the car park. Obviously our families were concerned about us too.

However, through it all we were able to keep morale up and support each other. The domestic staff – Peggy, Maureen, Marion, and the nursing assistants – Kathleen, Betty and so many others were key members of the team. Everyone pulled together.

They noticed when you had been working all day without a break and often Kathleen and Marion would come up to me when I was working with a patient and say: 'Sister, love, there's a wee tray in your office with something to eat.' They would have gone out to the shops to buy salad and fruit. They were so kind and generous.

Everyone would help the domestics. There were large dividing units between each bed in the main ward which needed to be moved out each morning so the ward could be cleaned. The consultants and nursing staff would assist the domestics in moving these and any other chores they required help with.

The technicians Jim and Brian were also important members of the team. They worked hard and kept things working. **"**

Broken images

"Four am. The dark hour. The hour before day begins and the time when the sick go quietly to their maker. The hour when the restless awake from their disturbed sleep and look out over a lonely city. A time for drinking coffee. A time for thinking of the past and people that you almost knew.

Four am. A time for broken images to start playing in my mind. Once more I can hear the screams and can feel the confusion the day they came in from the bookies' shop. Young fellas. Old. Gunshot wounds all spurting red.

Metal trolleys clanging through swinging doors. Weeping mothers comforting widows, not knowing of their own. Relatives being ushered into a quiet room with tea and the words: "We are doing the best we can." Knowing our best was never going to be good enough.

The shouts. The tears. The terror. Feet running. Voices raised.

'Get him into trauma quick.'
'What happened?'
'How many wounds?'
'Lift him on the table on the count of three.'
'Check for exit wounds.'
'Get another line into him.'
'Did anyone get a BP yet?'
'Any bleeders? Get the monitor on him. Put a bag of Hartman's up. Squeeze in those fluids.'
'Check the femoral pulse. Any BP yet?'

The heavy cloying smell of blood clogging the air. My shoes stained red. Expert hands cutting cloth from bone. Seconds of the Golden Hour ticking away. Sixty minutes to save a soul before time conspires against you. Frantic hands working desperately. Uniformed police with their raised guns and walkie-talkies. And through it all the cries of a woman. 'Has anyone seen my son?'

He held my hand. I could see the fear in his eyes.
He knew.
I knew. He kept his eyes on me. I kept my eyes on him.
He squeezed my hand, then the pressure of his hand on
mine lessened and fell away. He was 15.

Later outside the doors of trauma a woman grabbed
my arm.
'Have you seen my son?'
The hope. The fear.
She had his eyes.

Another day. The sound of a woman screaming:
'My legs. My legs.'
In a car somewhere.
In a car ripped apart by a bomb.
In a car somewhere...

Another day, two teenagers were brought in:
'I got two.'
'Only two? I got four. Knees and elbows. What did you
get? Ankles?'
'Yeah, you should have seen your face when they asked
you to lie down.'

They were given a time. They were told to be there.
They had a drink – for Dutch courage they said. They
turned up at the alley, on time. They turned their heads
away when the guns came out. They laughed when the
gun was placed at the back of their knees. They stopped
laughing when the gun went off:
Once. Twice. Three times. Four.
They were left with a limp... They were joyriders.

One time I held a man's hand after he was shot.
He was lucky.
His two friends were not.

'I'll always hear those footsteps,' he said. 'The only
sound I will ever hear again is the sound of those

footsteps searching for me. They knew I was there. They knew I was hiding. And those footsteps, they sounded so calm. No hurry at all. The gunman was taking his time, like. I could hear it in his footsteps. And he was searching for me. I held my breath and closed my eyes.'

More snapshots in the mind...

A taxi driver's fare turning to wave goodbye and watching as the taxi explodes.

Visiting a young lad in the community. Him cracking jokes. His mother fondly raising her eyes upwards. 'He's a torture that one. A real wee torture. He has me tortured.' She said still smiling, petting his hand. Real proud of him. You could see it in her eyes.

The construction of steel around his bed was the prison he couldn't escape from. Shot in the spine. Paralysed. Age? In his early twenties.

Two lads out for a drink. A night's craic. It was a good night until they stumbled into a sectarian crowd. They tried to run. They did run. They ran fast. They ran fast into a car. One dead. One not. They were still in their teens.

It's coming close to four in the morning again and more broken images in my head begin playing. And although I put those broken pieces together, I can never make sense of it. "

Martelle McPartland

Major incidents 1990-1999

"When I closed my eyes there was re-run after re-run of the devastation and cries of pain and grief."

A Health Visitor helping out in casualty

Shankill Road bomb, 1993

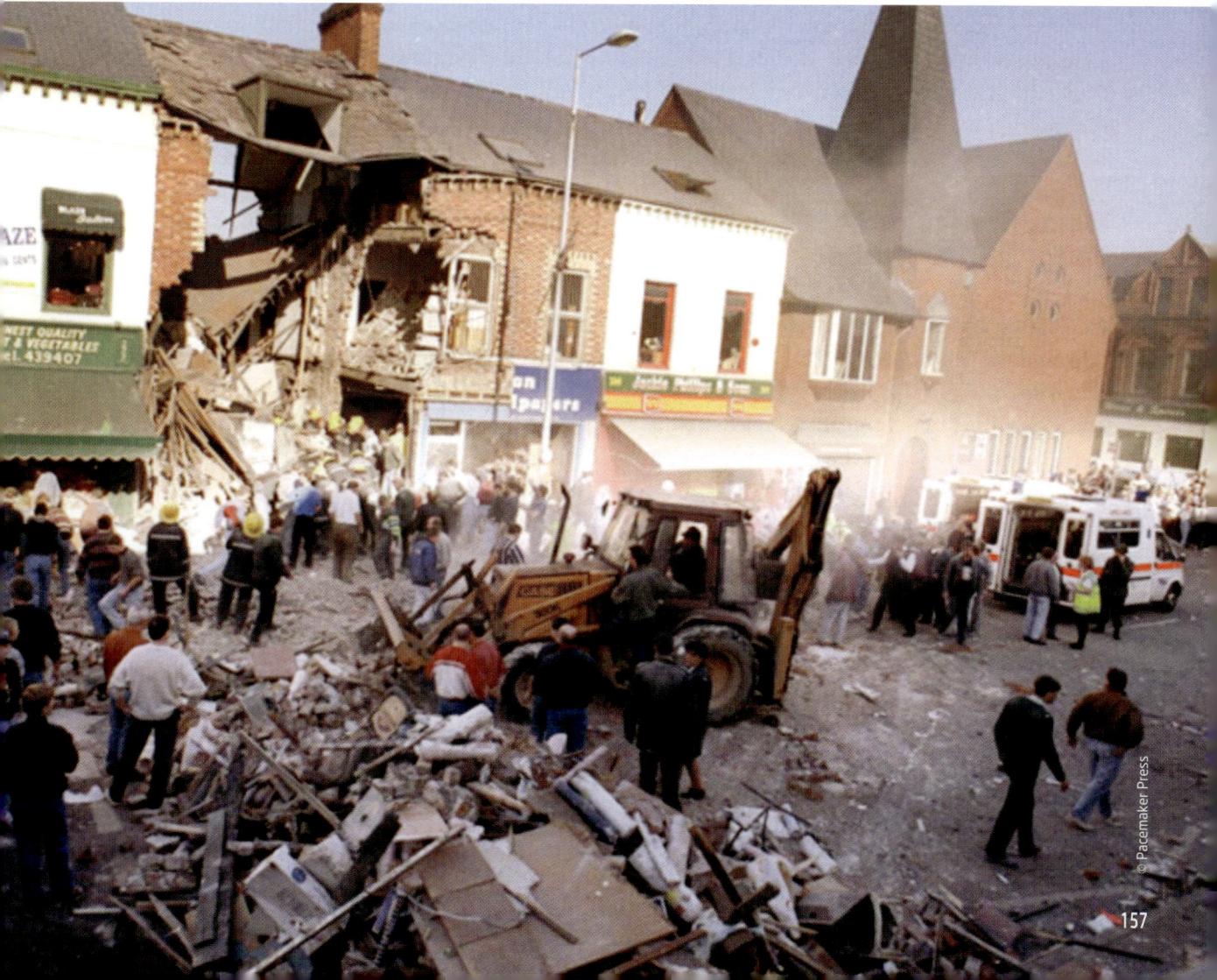

© Pacemaker Press

157

1990-1999
Deaths 530
Injured 10,811

31 August 1994 –
first IRA ceasefire

20 July 1997 –
second IRA ceasefire

10 April 1998 –
Good Friday or Belfast Agreement

The early months of 1992 witnessed increased sectarian violence. Political talks involving all parties had begun and developed at a slow pace. Eventually there were signs of hope for a cessation in violence. The Good Friday or Belfast Agreement was the breakthrough that started the Peace Process.

Memories from the Mater in the 1990s

"I started working in the Mater Hospital casualty in 1990. The department was separate from the main building, which meant to get patients to the ward they were wheeled outside in the rain, hail or snow. The entrance to the resuscitation unit was via the main waiting area, which meant the patients waiting to be seen had a great view of all the 'excitement' that was going on. Not surprisingly, we weren't asked too often how long the waiting time was or why they had to be seen. The reasons were evident before their very eyes.

We moved to a new department in 1991. At this time there was increased tension in the local community and often there was a tangible atmosphere in the department. We all knew something was going to happen, but we just didn't know what or when. Night duty was particularly eerie. Very few people happened to be wandering about North Belfast after dark in those days, so we knew that anyone who came in through our doors was there for a very good reason.

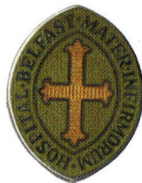

I recall one particular evening when a well-known paramilitary was in the department with some of his 'minders'. A few minutes after they left we got a shout from reception to say that a taxi driver had been shot just outside the department. He had been called to casualty to pick up a fare. He thought it was safe to come to the Mater. At that time there were a number of taxi men who were randomly shot across the city. We immediately took the taxi driver into resuscitation and began working on him. Thankfully he survived.

I met him a number of years later when he attended the Mater again. When I recognised him he told me that following the shooting incident he had suffered from severe depression and struggled to work again.

In the Mater casualty, everyone from across the community attended for treatment. We regularly had patients from the Loyalist Shankill and Tiger's Bay areas, and from the Nationalist New Lodge and Ardoyne. This was in itself a challenge to manage. If you were aware that there were members from different factions waiting to be seen, you tried to get one group seen and treated as quickly as possible to avoid the possibility of confrontation in the waiting room. On occasions things would 'kick off' and there would be trouble between groups. This resulted in an immediate call to North Queen Street Police Station. Thankfully the police were always very responsive.

I recall one incident when a young soldier had been brought in the back of an army jeep. He had been shot in the neck. We desperately tried to cut off his protective clothing to start resuscitation. I remember the sense of urgency amongst the team. Sadly he died despite all our efforts to resuscitate him.

His colleagues, not surprisingly, were devastated. However they still had to remain alert to the potential threat to themselves. I remember collecting the soldier's belongings together and seeing his dog tags. I had never seen these before and I suppose at that time I didn't really understand the significance.

Regardless of his profession, he was someone's son, brother, husband or father; like every other man who had died in that room.

In the Mater Hospital there was always a real sense of camaraderie, everyone knew each other, and despite the tension in the community around us, we all worked extremely well together as a team. There was always plenty of 'craic' and humour on night duty, when you knew there wouldn't be too many patients coming through the door. I suppose this was our way of coping to try to deal with some of the tragic situations we witnessed.**"**

Musgrave Park Hospital, Belfast Bomb, 2 November 1991

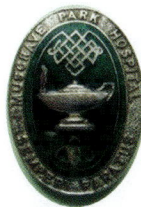

A bomb exploded at the military wing of Musgrave Park Hospital killing two soldiers and injuring 18.

Flashback to World War Two
"I was on night duty in the spinal cord injuries unit the Saturday following the bomb blast at the hospital. I was told we were to have patients transferred from the orthopaedics ward. All the patients were upset and it took a while to settle them.

One elderly man in particular was very agitated and I spent some time trying to reassure him. He couldn't sleep and kept asking me why I was walking about. At one point I was looking out the window, and he asked me if I was watching out for bombers.

I tried to reassure him that there would be no more bombs. I sat with him for a while until he was calmer and I thought he would settle. A short time later he called me and asked if I knew whether the Germans were coming back and if we would be safe in the shelter. I realised that he was convinced that we were in an air-raid shelter and were waiting on the night raid from German aircraft.

It was a difficult shift that evening following the bombing. The distress of all the patients was difficult to cope with while trying to be calm and reassuring. It was so sad to see how it had so badly affected that elderly man. It put him right back in World War Two.**"**

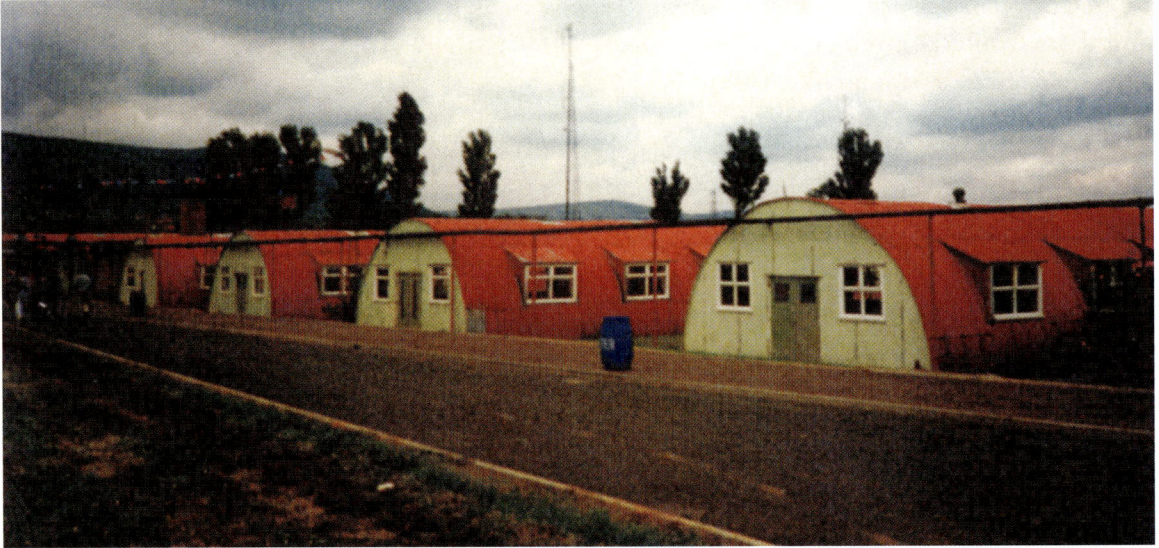

Musgrave Park Nissen huts

The day our ward was bombed

❝I was one of two ward sisters responsible for children with a variety of orthopaedic problems and complex syndromes. The patient group were children up to 18 years old. Our combined unit of two wards used to accommodate parents and carers who 'roomed in' to support their children.

On Friday 1 November 1991 a decision was made to relocate the children's wards from the World War Two Nissen huts to a refurbished ground floor unit in the main hospital known as Withers 2A and 2B. Nursing staff had reservations as the new accommodation was not complete. This was most apparent on the A ward, which was to accommodate the older children. It was decided to move the youngest patients first and those who could be discharged were sent home with medication and follow-up appointments. Seven patients and their parents transferred to the new ward.

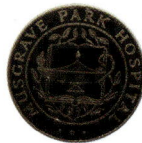

Arriving at work on 2 November I found the night staff apprehensive as during their shift they had observed a man loitering outside the unit. Following an extensive search by security no one had been found and it was assumed he must have been a taxi driver.

Later on that day there was a loud bang with a continuous ripping sound which appeared to come from the kitchen. The whole ward rattled. I looked outside and saw with horror the road erupting followed by the collapse of the adjacent building, which housed the military wing.

Aware that the bomb must have been planted in the basement area below our ward, our immediate priority was to assess our patients, their parents and staff, and then remove them to a place of safety, while remaining conscious of the risk of the building collapsing. Thankfully only one patient suffered minor harm and a father sustained a minor injury.

When you bombed our hospital...

Sir,
As the memory of the Musgrave Park Hospital bombing inevitably begins to fade, we — a group of nurses from the hospital on duty that day — can no longer remain silent.

Through your column, therefore, we would address not only those who bombed us, but all who use or support violence within our society for espoused political ends.

For the 20-plus years of this political conflict, thousands of people have been killed or injured. For the same period and long before, nurses here at Musgrave Park Hospital and at institutions all over Northern Ireland have treated the sick without question, without judgement, without prejudice.

The nurses who do this work come from all sides of the community, with varying political beliefs. We work together not by coercion, but by choice. We work together because we want to.

Yes, of course, we have our differences. But for us, because we have a common goal — our patients — cooperation and even reconciliation is reality.

Hospitals have always been seen as places of care, hope, comfort and acceptance. Yet you felt your politics allowed you to bomb us.

Is it now not time for you to ask yourselves, when your campaign has become so callous, for all the violence,

Readers' opinions are welcome on any subject. Send submissions to: Readers' Forum, The Irish News, 113-117 Donegall Street, Belfast, BT1 2GE; or fax them to (0232) 231282. All letters must be accompanied by the name and address of the author. Where possible they should be typed and on one side of the page.

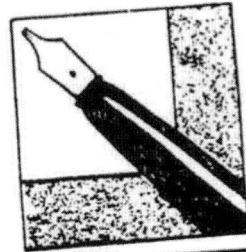

what have you achieved? How closer are you to your aims?

Surely, no matter what your aims, or who you claim to be a "legitimate target," there can be no justification for attacking those least able to defend themselves...the sick, the old and the young. All of these you attacked when you bombed our hospital.

Maybe the very place you attacked and the people in it can provide a clue as to how our problem here in Northern Ireland may advance towards solution. Many of our patients come to hospital with serious debilitating problems which severely disrupt their daily lives. Their problems must be accurately diagnosed — sometimes, a lengthy and difficult procedure.

For the problem to be cured, often a long, sometimes painful, period of treatment is started. Frequently, this treatment involves patients returning to hospital again and again. But they do this; they continue with their treatment because their desire for a cure is greater than the pain or inconvenience endured in its attainment.

After 20 years of destruction, do you have the courage to re-examine your methods? Is there another way to a solution?

In conclusion, we want the people of Northern Ireland to know that, no matter who you are, if you need our help, the nurses of Musgrave Park Hospital will give it without question. Your political affiliation does not matter to us; the fact that you are ill does.

Yours,
A Group of Nurses,
Musgrave Park Hospital

Rows at jail could curb help activities

Sir,
Recently, there have been incidents of violence, inside and outside Crumlin Road Prison, involving prisoners'

A major concern was the welfare of the military personnel, particularly as we knew how many would have been watching television coverage of the World Cup rugby final between England and Australia that afternoon. We knew the recreation room was in the collapsed part of the building and we set up an emergency field hospital adjacent to the military wing.

Dr Denis Connolly, a consultant anaesthetist who happened to be in our ward, assisted with the treatment of casualties. Two soldiers had been killed in the blast and ten others suffered injuries.

Looking back, I am always amazed that calmness, compassion and competence overcame chaos and confusion. We had to put aside our utter disbelief that a children's ward had been used to access and facilitate the bombing of the military wing, with no regard for the danger to which this exposed other patients. This incident was to prove to be an all-time low in a catalogue of events depicting man's inhumanity to man.

A group of us as nurses wrote an open letter to the papers appealing to the bombers to stop. 🙿

Shootings at Sean Graham's Bookmakers, Ormeau Road, 5 February 1992

Five civilians were killed, including a 15 year old, and nine were wounded in a gun attack in a bookmaker's shop in Belfast on a busy Wednesday afternoon.

Gunshot wounds

❝I can remember clearly the afternoon of the shooting on the Ormeau Road. Fortunately for us, it was an afternoon when there were no theatre lists.

We received a number of casualties to Belfast City Hospital, and I can remember dealing with a 15-year-old boy who had multiple gunshot wounds. Despite our efforts, he died in my care.

This image was to remain with me for the rest of my life. I can still see his family in the trauma room lifting the sheet off his body to see the wounds.❞

Shankill Road Bomb, 23 October 1993

Ten people were killed when a bomb exploded in a fish shop. A further 57 people were injured.

First experience at Mater Hospital A&E

❝As a newly qualified Staff Nurse of 21, I had landed a temporary post in the Mater accident and emergency department in October 1993. Returning from a tea break a colleague came around the corner shouting: 'Quick, there has been a bomb on the Shankill.'

I remember thinking 'Oh dear God – what does that mean for us?' I didn't hear the bomb go off so I wasn't sure if it was a big or small blast. I was very naive.

I was immediately assigned to resuscitation with a senior nurse. I was the most junior staff nurse in the department and had zero training for this situation. Before I could think anymore I had gloved up and our first victims had arrived.

I followed everything the senior nurse did or told me to do. I watched her start to cut clothes off our first patient and I just copied her. She cut one leg of the trousers and I cut the other. We worked simultaneously. One patient didn't look very good. He had a bad head injury, was unconscious and not breathing properly.

I glanced across the room as I couldn't ignore the screams coming from another patient. He looked like his head had been dipped in red paint and I remember with horror how much pain he must have been suffering to squeal in that way.

Another patient was wheeled in on an ambulance trolley. It looked like a small body and I thought: 'Where the hell are we going to put him? And I hope they don't ask me to look after him on my own because I won't know what to do.'

Then he was taken away. I think he was a child. I think he was dead.

After our patient was transferred to the Royal intensive care unit I was assigned to level two where the 'walk in' patients arrived – though just because they were walk in did not mean they were not seriously injured. I ran up to level two, despite being reluctant to leave A&E.

When I arrived there I found people everywhere screaming, crying and wandering around with disbelief in their eyes. There were bloodied heads, faces and limbs. I remember seeing a girl with blonde hair with a bad head wound and thinking she was probably the same age as me.

I worked with a medical consultant who had been called in from home to help. He was a little uncertain about tetanus cover, how to close head wounds, whether to use sutures or staples and when they should be removed. I felt pretty confident in advising him in this area.

Eventually the patients stopped coming and I was summoned back to A&E. I couldn't believe it – there were no patients. They had all gone!

We had a short de-briefing on the events with the A&E consultant who praised us highly. Even then I wasn't sure if I had made much of a difference. It was a Saturday and yet every senior manager and director in the Mater was standing in the A&E department, though it was eerily quiet now.

The consultant I had worked with was pointing at me and I could hear him saying how well I had worked and how I had kept him right about the patients' treatments. I felt very embarrassed and I couldn't believe I was getting praise from a consultant – an event unheard of throughout my training.

I hadn't realised I was well over my shift and eventually the charge nurse said I could go home though, to be honest, I didn't want to leave. I was afraid another catastrophe could happen and I wanted to be on hand to help.

It was only when I got home and the TV was on in the living room that I was able to watch the atrocity of that day unfold. Seeing it from the public's perspective I could absorb the seriousness of it all.

Watching the ambulance crews I had grown to know in my short time in casualty, standing in the rubble lifting bricks trying to rescue people, I couldn't comprehend the extent of the event I had just taken part in and how so many people had been affected.

On the Monday morning I was summoned by the Director of Nursing and offered a permanent post on the back of my performance that Saturday. I couldn't believe it! I accepted, though it felt bitter sweet that something good could come out of an event that caused so much suffering to the victims and their families.

I still work in A&E as a senior sister and often wonder how differently I would react as the nurse in charge if I received a call from ambulance control with a similar scenario. I now have the experience and the training, and feel privileged to have been part of something that was so significant But I wouldn't wish to be involved in anything like it ever again. **"**

The two "sides" at close quarters

"I was a staff nurse on ward 37 in the Royal when the Shankill bombing took place. I was working nights alongside another staff nurse and an auxiliary nurse. It was an extraordinary night for all of us. The ward was packed with wounded, distressed, traumatised people from all walks of life who just happened to be in the wrong place at the wrong time.

The strangest thing was that the relatives of the boy who planted the bomb were sitting beside the relatives of the wounded, totally oblivious to each other until a nurse made the discovery and quickly sorted out new waiting areas. We were all stunned that it was not discovered sooner, or worse, that the relatives had made the connection themselves.

Cups of tea had been handed out all night and our auxiliary would take a fit of the giggles every time she thought about the 'tea party' at the doors. I always thought you needed a strange sense of humour to get you through nursing and we certainly developed one that night.**"**

Reflections on the Shankill bomb

"On that day we never questioned who we cared for or why they were in hospital. They were our patients, not bombers or innocent bystanders, just our patients.

I think this was what we had to do to be able to care for everyone who came through the doors. Everyone received the care they needed that night based on their injuries, not their religious or their political persuasion. It was a mark of our training that we could step up to the challenge time after time without ever thinking of anything other than providing the care we were trained to give. Well done to the teachers who made us what we are!**"**

Coping with stress

"Some stories we as nurses heard told in the community were emotionally draining – we were traumatised by what people had to endure. All of us were probably under stress and didn't know it."

Community Psychiatric Nurse

A light-hearted moment in the snow

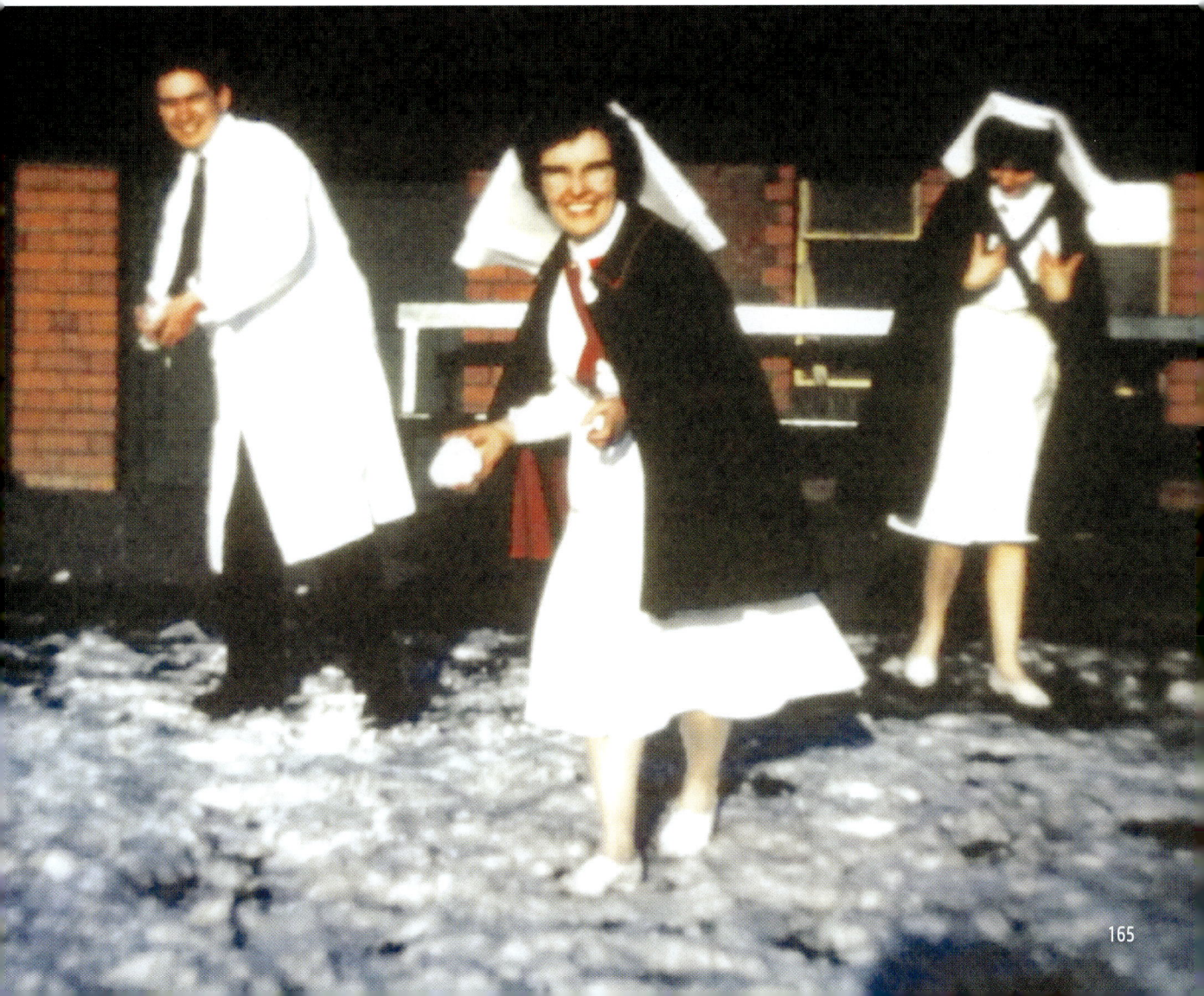

Keeping spirits up

"We just got on with it." That was the most frequent comment from nurses who told their story. Many noted there was no counselling on offer to staff for the experiences they had to endure, often on a regular basis.

Although many nurses contributed to this book, others who, although glad that these accounts were being recorded, did not feel able to tell their story. Many had purposely tried to forget the horrific experiences that they witnessed some 30 to 40 years ago.

They could not speak about La Mon. The Enniskillen and Omagh bombs were, for some, too recent to discuss. For these nurses events of those days are indelibly ingrained in their minds and they still overwhelm them and tears flow.

Nurses emphasised how much they relied on each other's companionship and informal "chats" over a cuppa, either in their workplace or in the nurses' home.

Impromptu tea parties were a common feature in some areas to provide relief. Casualty Sister Kate O'Hanlon at the Royal Victoria Hospital had a reputation for celebrating any birthday or anniversary.

She also organised "casualty revues", social outings and sports events to help promote morale and team work and provide some fun in the unit. It was obligatory for all staff to become involved.

"One of the ways in which casualty staff kept their spirits up was to occasionally mount some entertainment. Any excuse would do, and if there was no one being promoted, getting married or leaving, then an occasional 'revue' would be organised."
Casualty Staff Nurse

Ward activities were also arranged by respiratory and intensive care unit staff.

"However, we also enjoyed ourselves too. We had regular hockey matches against the A&E staff; in the summertime we had barbeques with the best of steaks, and strawberries and cream!

At Christmas my father would bone a turkey and cook it for me to bring in with salads for Christmas lunch. We had a party every Christmas morning when the medical staff and their families came in for refreshments. There were dinners during the year, especially if staff were moving on to new posts. There was a real sense of family among us all. We supported each other through the good times as well as the difficult times. That's what made it all so special.**

A cancelled night out

"During December in the late 1970s, nights out with colleagues were deemed unsafe. Not to be deterred, Miss Mary McGrane, Nursing Officer for ICU, A&E outpatients and OT, arranged an evening get-together in the OT area at Craigavon Area Hospital. As was the fashion, nursing staff arrived wearing long dresses and entered via the A&E entrance.

It soon became clear that an incident had occurred. Led by Sister Joan Heaney, staff hitched up their long dresses, put on plastic aprons and assisted where needed. 🙶

Not only was the effect of trauma on health service staff not identified in the early years of the Troubles, but the mental health effects on patients caught up in atrocities was also not recognised or addressed at first. The physical care of wounds was well attended to, but the psychological needs of the long-term effects associated with traumatic experiences, such as loss of limbs, severe physical disability or just having survived a major incident were not fully acknowledged. "You were lucky to be alive!"

"I worked as a community psychiatric nurse, it really annoyed me when I would hear on the radio that a family had been held up for so many hours but were not injured. It just showed how nobody was grasping the psychological impact that this would have on a family."
Community Psychiatric Nurse

Clifton Street Day Hospital

🙶I was working at this unit, which was for people who had experienced a range of mental health problems, in February 1970. My work in West Belfast gave me a chance to assess the effects of the riots on the patients referred to the Day Hospital.

I undertook a study of 140 patients from February to the end of September 1970 who had been admitted to the unit as a result of barricades, burning, intimidation and shooting. A total of 16 of the patients were admitted due to stress. Symptoms experienced were insomnia, anorexia, inability to cope, anxiety, depression, fear, anger, fear of going out. One of the patient's sons had been shot dead and she blamed herself as she had taken him into his bedroom for safety.

The unemployed were more likely to develop symptoms in these conditions. Under the stress of a riot, those with a psychiatric history tend to have a recurrence of their previous illness.

Although the Peace Line separated the patients in the community, they socialised well in hospital and did not show any signs of hostility towards each other. 🙶

Psychological trauma

🙶I remember one young man who lost both legs in an Ulster Volunteer Force bomb blast at the Glen Inn in 1976. His wounds were heavily contaminated, and for a long time he was toxic and confused. After he stabilised I thought of getting him to read Alf McCreary's book 'Survivors', which described the experience of earlier Troubles amputees.

My intervention was instinctive rather than rational. And I didn't ask anyone's permission. In that era and since, second-year staff nurses weren't supposed to show any startling initiative. I was hesitant about my offer: what if details of the road ahead were to plunge the patient into depression? But I needn't have worried. The young man

www.belfasttelegraph.co.uk

DAY TWO: The Catholic man caught in a UVF bomb who felt he was left to fend for himself

VICTIMS
What they really think

I said to the nurse: "I've lost my legs, haven't I?" I accepted it instantly. I had no choice. I was 18 years of age and lucky to be alive

Divorced father-of-four Mark Kelly MBE (right), was left a double amputee after a UVF bomb attack on the Glen Inn, Glengormley, on the night of Saturday, August 28, 1976. The 48-year-old Catholic tells **Gráinne McCarry** how he received no support in coping with the emotional fall-out of his injuries. He says:

> I had stopped at the Glen Inn to have a drink with a few friends to celebrate scoring three goals in a Gaelic football match

Mark Kelly - Belfast Telegraph

seized Survivors with obvious enthusiasm, and fixed his gaze on the title. 'I'm a survivor!' he proclaimed, and began to read. Thirty one years later, I was astonished to see this episode featured in a Belfast newspaper. 'There was no counselling, no support, no guidance. You had to fend for yourself. I was so tired. The will to live had left me. A nurse gave me a copy of Alf McCreary's book, Survivors. It was very helpful to me when I was recovering… the words in that book were really the only emotional support that I got.' (Mark Kelly, Belfast Telegraph, 13 February 2007).

After the ceasefire

"For a minute I thought I was going to lose control of the whole situation for there were people so badly injured. It was terrible to think that as a qualified nurse you might not be in control of the situation."

Staff Nurse

Omagh bomb, Main Street, 1998

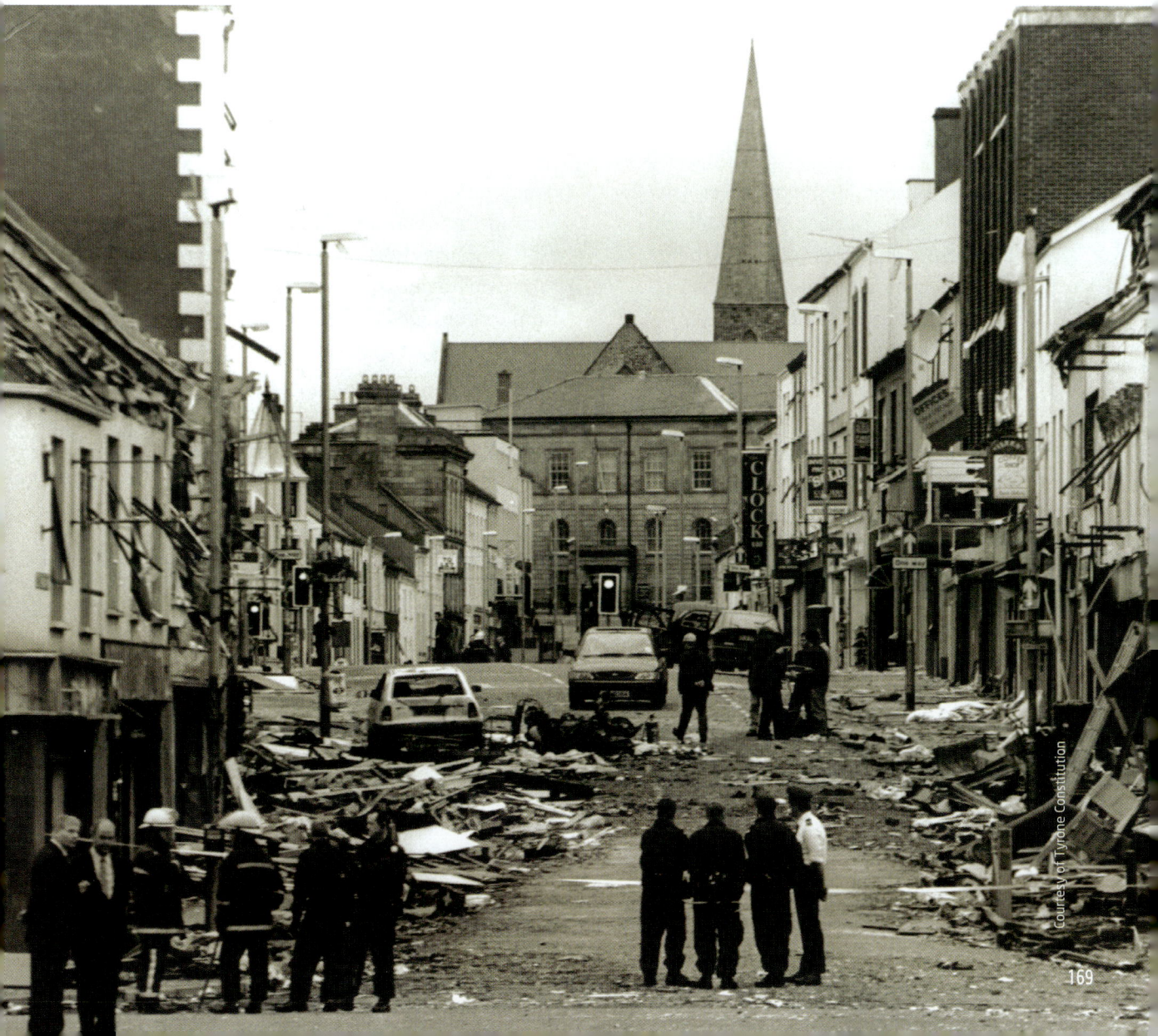

Courtesy of Tyrone Constitution

Sadly, tragedy exploded back onto the streets when paramilitary dissidents detonated a bomb in Omagh, County Tyrone killing 29 people as well as unborn twins.

There were more than 220 casualties, some with major and life-threatening injuries. The Omagh bomb was the worst single atrocity of the Troubles, causing the greatest number of deaths and injuries. All were civilians.

Omagh bombing, 15 August 1998

"On that Saturday at 3.04pm, a terrorist car bomb exploded in Market Street, Omagh. Whilst warning had been given by the perpetrators, they had not been clear in stating the location of their device, and vaguely referred to the local courthouse as being their target.

With this in mind the police had evacuated the area and imposed a cordon of four hundred yards, beyond which many of those in the town were waiting patiently in the hope of a 'false alarm' and a return to their shopping and socialising.

Consequently the narrow street lined on either side by busy shops was packed with men, women and children. They were oblivious to the chilling fact that one of the cars in their midst, on which some of them leant, contained the bomb.

The explosion led to the deaths of 29 people and unborn twins. Twenty six families were bereaved, three from the Irish Republic, two in Spain and 20 from the locality of Omagh. Tragically another person died in a traffic collision with an ambulance transferring one of the injured to hospital. More than 370 people were injured and were admitted to hospital or attended for treatment as a result of the explosion. Of this number, 60 were significantly or seriously injured. At the inquest it was revealed that the street was cleared of all casualties by 3.40pm.

The bombing ranks as one of the most brutal attacks associated with the current phase of Troubles in Ireland. The bomb occurred at a time of supposed peace. Indeed the death toll is the highest for any single incident. Many have been exposed to powerful images, sounds and smells of human carnage and suffering which may have significant psychological implications.

The high number of casualties included elderly people, women and children as well as visitors from the Republic of Ireland and Spain. A number of staff had relatives killed or injured and many knew the victims.

That day I was playing a football match with Omagh Hospitals Football Club. When we heard the explosion we continued playing, as we did not know the extent of the tragedy. When news filtered through of the dead and injured, those of us who work in the health service rushed to Tyrone County Hospital. But first I went home to check my family were okay. Thank God they had gone to the cinema.

What I saw in the hospital will remain with me for the rest of my life, as it will for so many others. Nurses, doctors, the ambulance service, the police, radiologists, the clergy, social workers, managers, clerical staff, porters, lab technicians, laundry, domestic and catering staff, the army, voluntary agencies and the public all tried to work together to save lives, comfort relatives and look after each other.

I was listening to people's concerns and their enquiries. Many were desperately looking for family, relatives and friends who were missing, and as each hour passed, the realisation began to dawn that they might be seriously injured or dead. I arrived one hour after the bomb.

Before the explosion there were two nurses and one doctor on duty in the A&E department. It was quiet. The nurses heard the explosion but like so many others believed at that time that there was only property damage.

Within minutes, and before additional staff could be mustered, scores of casualties began arriving at Tyrone County Hospital. Patients arrived by bus, ambulance, taxi, private car, vans and on foot. Staff quickly converged on the hospital after hearing of the bomb and the level of carnage, to offer what assistance and support they could. A radio and TV appeal was launched for more staff.

The first casualty to arrive was a baby carried in by a member of the public. He handed the child to the nurse. Here is what she said on a radio interview:

'The baby was off-colour. I needed an anaesthetist, which I got right away, to see to the baby. We don't know who the baby is, but I looked after this baby and... more patients were coming into casualty. I knew I would be distracted if I looked either way and ambu-bagged the baby but I knew – we had lost the fight for its life. But I hugged it and I kissed it and I hope the parents know that I took care of it in whatever way I could and then after that I put it aside gently and carried on with the next casualty which was a young boy on a trolley.'

Casualties were all over the place and each one seemed worse than the other. For one junior nurse the worst thing for her was the blood everywhere, from the waiting room to the theatre. For many staff the most difficult part in the initial stages was not knowing if their family, relations and friends were involved in the bombing. Again quoting another nurse:

'I was numbed at the beginning. Then I thought, my own girls could be in this somewhere, because I had two daughters in the town. I knew that they were going to be down there where the bomb had exploded as they were shopping for jeans.

And all the time in the back of my mind I was thinking, are they going to be there, you know, who am I going to meet next – it could be them and my feelings were totally mixed up and yet, you just had to carry on and deal with the people who were so badly injured.

And then late on some of the girls rang from home. They had managed to get through and I felt reassured that they were okay, and I felt guilty as well, you know, that I had come off unscathed myself and there were so many people that were so badly injured and it could well have been me or mine. They were peoples' relatives.'

A sense of being overwhelmed was also evident with many nurses. As one nurse put it:

'...the patients were screaming in pain, "help me, help me". They weren't in ones or twos, they were in twenties and thirties.

After triage and stabilisation patients were either kept or transferred to other hospitals and eventually, after working late into the night, things began to settle. I left the hospital late that night, having done what I could but feeling I could have done more. I had little sleep that night. Every time I closed my eyes, one horrible image was replaced by another, even worse.

In the days and weeks following the bomb staff worked extra shifts to provide continuous care. I was initially involved in staff support.

On the Monday following the bomb, occupational health organised a meeting to co-ordinate a range of support services for staff. This support included organising both group and individual sessions for staff to talk to trained professionals. Other groups also became involved in support such as the Royal College of Nursing, the WAVE Trauma Centre, Victim Support and the Staff Support Network from Belfast. However, there was very little uptake on these services.'

The occupational doctor for the trust explained:

'What I've noticed in the first couple of weeks is that staff have responded beyond what you would think was humanly possible. So clearly, there is a phase of tiredness that all staff will feel.

The one thing that an academic would tell you, and I am not an academic in this field, is that there will be a protective numbness for a number of staff, and perhaps it would be wrong to provoke, poke or require them to undergo any complex form of treatment or counselling at this stage.

But, we must be prepared that at some stage, we must be alert to these people, we must have available to them, in their timescale, the various forms of support or whatever help they need.'

Another nurse described her feelings:

'I was numb, I cried... I went over how I had coped myself and I felt that I had coped inadequately, you know, I felt I hadn't done enough for the people that were injured. I felt awful.

I didn't sleep that night nor for a few nights afterwards and even yet there are nights I wake up with flashbacks of things that were coming.'

Others felt sadness, grief, depression, anxiety, dread and fear, rage, shame. For some it was too much to return to the hospital, as there were reminders of the tragedy everywhere.

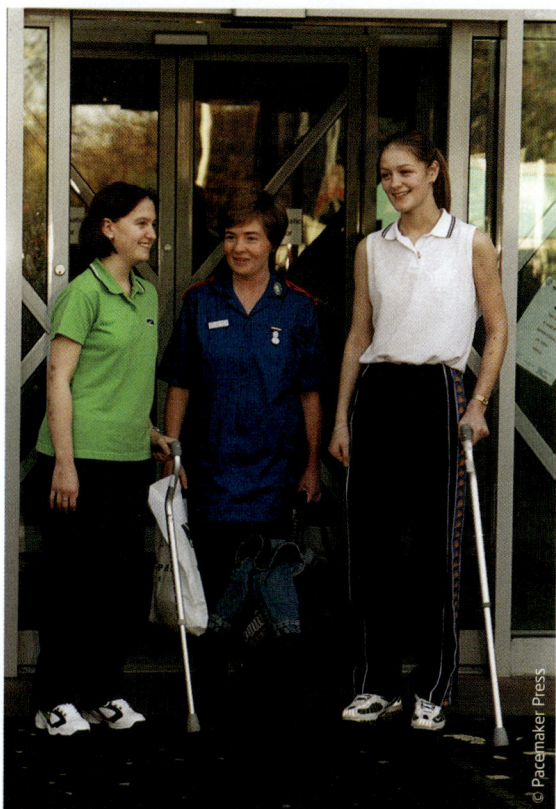
Omagh bomb victims, 1998

One nurse spoke of the difficulty staff's families often had to comprehend what they had been through:

'My family are not of any medical or nursing background, other than myself. So it's difficult for them to understand. Right enough they put their arms around me, but I don't think they know it was terrible and they feel terrible. But to work in the situation, I don't think they really feel they understand what it's like.'

Another nurse commented:

'I said at that time I didn't feel the need for counselling because I think just talking to colleagues who had been there and went through the same thing was enough counselling. Everybody is different. You know I'm sure there are people that felt the need of counselling straight off. I might well have to avail myself of counselling. It is just the flashbacks I keep getting. I don't know how to cope with it, how long it's going to go on for. You keep going over in your mind: is there something more you could have done? And it is just a matter of talking through it, you know? There's nothing can really take it away, unless... I think talking definitely does help.'

Avoidance was a big issue. Difficulties in falling or staying asleep, irritability or outbursts of anger, difficulty in concentrating were all evident. Also people had persistent headaches and other somatic complaints, such as backache and gastrointestinal distress. Some staff also talked of personal relationships being affected.

In the longer term some nurses were said to be suffering from post-traumatic stress disorder, which includes intrusive thoughts, avoidance behaviours and increased awareness. Other nurses have suffered depression and suicidal tendencies, panic attacks and over-reliance on alcohol.

Some nurses did take up the offer of counselling when provided by the RCN. But for most nurses the best support came from colleagues. Everyone is different and everybody reacts differently to trauma. We all have our own coping strategies.

We will all remember this day for the rest of our lives. **"**

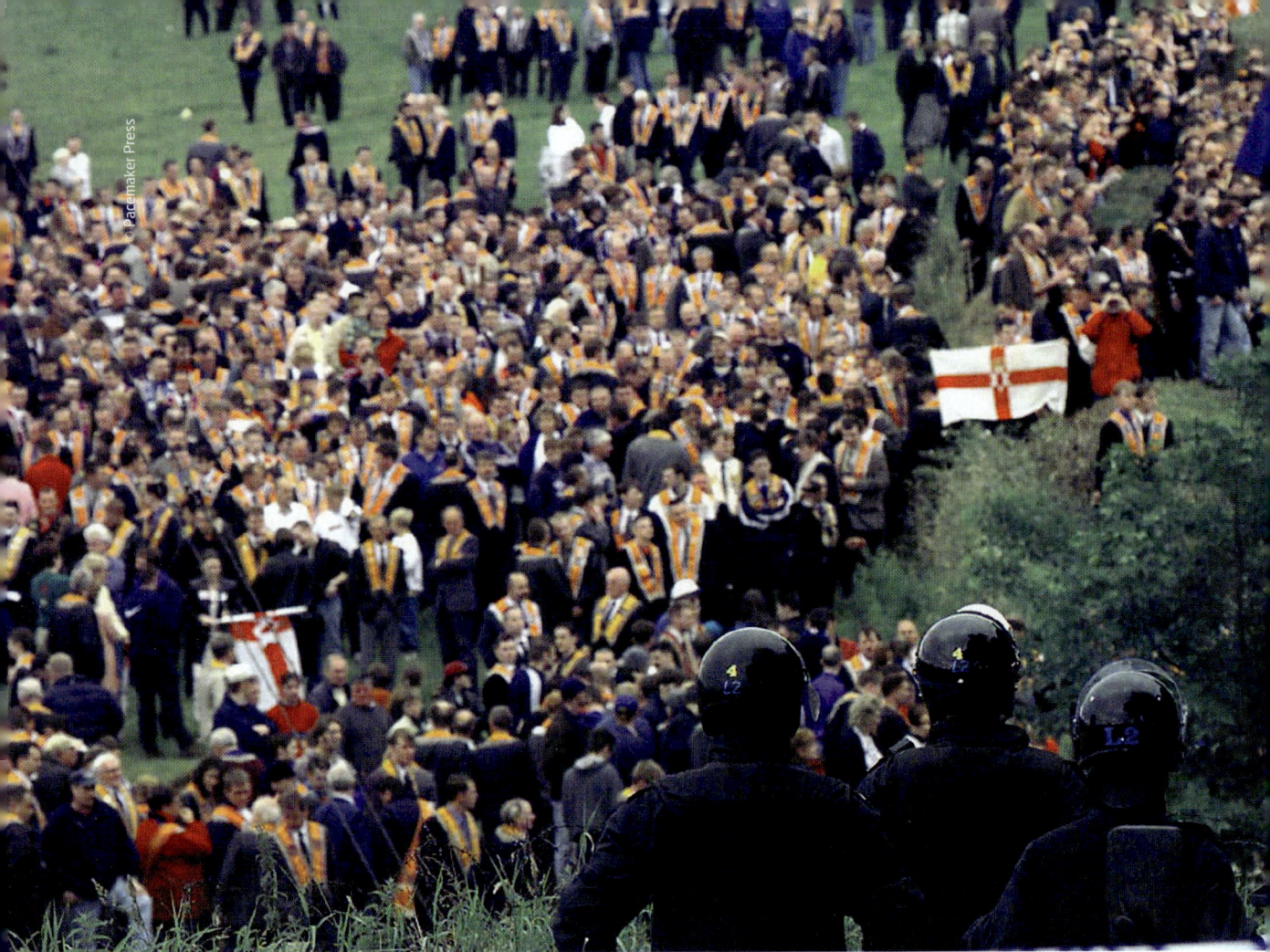

Drumcree stand-off, 1998

Drumcree Orange Order July Parades 1995-1998

For the duration of the Troubles hospitals had remained on high alert, continually reviewing their major disaster plans based on the experiences of the previous atrocity. In contrast, the annual Drumcree conflict became an anticipated problem.

The following account shows the planning involved. To a lesser degree the same process was practised by other hospitals and community units across the province as they prepared for this contentious parade.

"In April 1998 staff at Craigavon Hospital began preparations for potential major violence during the last week in June and the first week of July.

Over the previous four years civil disturbances had erupted as a result of the banning of the annual Orange Order parade to Drumcree Church, Portadown, which was usually held on the first Sunday in July. The whole of Northern Ireland was affected, but Craigavon was at the eye of the storm.

The level of violence and civil unrest greatly increased over this period.

Official statistics from this two weeks in 1998 showed that there were 25 shootings, 56 bombings, 391 incidents of intimidation, 642 petrol bombs thrown, 178 hijackings, 884 properties damaged, 1,372 unofficial road blocks reported and 1,200 plastic-baton rounds fired. This was significantly down on the previous three years!

The situation was likely to be drawn out over at least two weeks, which resulted in the hospital having to remain in a prolonged state of preparedness. The impact this had on the staff was significant. The psychological and emotional impact of anticipating, expecting and waiting for the inevitable major incident to occur was great.

When the inevitable finally happened, casualties needed to be segregated. When the injured from rival groups arrive in A&E, the site of the rioting is simply transferred to the casualty department.

Planning
Planning began two months in advance. The Major Incident Working Group involved senior clinicians and trust management. Their involvement was essential. The chief executive played an active role and his visibility was much appreciated.

In all the years of Drumcree, transportation to and from work for hospital and community staff had been hazardous. All trust staff were given security passes to help them get through any unofficial roadblocks set up by protestors around the countryside.

The plan involved setting up a second emergency room, segregated from the main A&E, with four resuscitation beds in the theatre and recovery area. In the past, there had been serious rioting when casualties arrived, the department becoming a volatile and dangerous place for staff and patients; every effort had to be made to minimise the threat of violence.

Recovery and theatres
The sisters in the recovery/high dependency unit were responsible for organising staffing and equipping the temporary unit. Three senior A&E staff rotated on a 24-hour basis, complementing the rota for recovery and theatre staff. There were four further beds which could be used at short notice for resuscitation if required.

Military casualties were assigned a dedicated route into the second emergency room. This was tested by military personnel with temporary but clear signage and was found to be safe and effective. The least complicated option was to assign a special area for military casualties. Only seriously ill military patients came to this area. Arrangements were made for military medical teams to treat their own non-emergency casualties, so a 12-bed hospital was set up at the local army base to deal with minor injuries.

It was decided that no 'minor' injuries to police or army would come to A&E over this period of civil unrest. If there were more casualties than Craigavon could cope with, other hospitals had to be used.

On June 29 the Parades Commission announced its decision to prohibit the Drumcree Parade. The decision itself made no difference to the plan, but it did mean there was a greater potential for serious trouble from this day on. The first incidents of civil disturbance occurred almost immediately, with widespread hijacking of cars and buses.

Many staff chose to stay in the hospital student accommodation rather than travel and face the risk of hijacking or intimidation, so 30 rooms were made available for them.

All leave for A&E nurses and doctors was cancelled and they became part of a 24-hour rota with two nurses on call for A&E, with one senior A&E nurse, two recovery staff and one theatre nurse for the second emergency room. This was essential to maximise the team approach and make the best use of the specialist skills.

Ward activity was scaled down, with all major surgery – with the exception of emergencies and cancer cases – cancelled. This obviously had a knock-on effect on already prolonged waiting lists.

A&E senior nurses were authorised to admit patients directly to wards and a neighbouring trust, South Tyrone Hospital, offered assistance in the form of a nurse on call 24/7.

Stand off
In 1998, the situation worsened as the stand-off continued. There were over 30,000 protesters gathering at night with the possibility of over 100,000 people arriving by July 13. The tension in the community and sense of impending doom was reaching a crescendo. Thousands of extra troops were drafted in and we braced ourselves for what

might happen. On the worst nights of violence the plans were certainly tested, with plastic bullet, blast- and petrol-bomb injuries. This included a number of serious life- and limb-threatening injuries.

However, over in Ballymoney, an arson attack by Loyalists led to the death of three young brothers. The deaths were described by the police as sectarian murders and caused revulsion across the province and beyond. Although this happened in another part of Northern Ireland, it signalled an end to the main protests and hence the potential for serious violence diminished rapidly.

It is difficult to describe the feelings of staff when this happened. Many staff wept openly in despair and grief at such a senseless tragedy and there was a ghostly silence in the department for days. Ironically however, this despair was tinted with a sense of relief around our own circumstances, that is, our very worst fears had not materialised

Over the four years of Drumcree, the last week in June and the first week in July was an extremely challenging time for everybody in Northern Ireland and for emergency and community nurses in particular. The challenges presented to us were evident, but the professionalism of those involved was exceptional. As challenging as it was, this unique experience proved incredibly valuable to nursing staff as an exercise in building, strengthening and developing relationships and resilience in the face of fear and despair. Nurses proved once again that they had the experience and skills to make a difference during such difficult times.**"**

Peacetime

❝I worked as a community nurse in North and West Belfast for more than 30 years from 1980. By the time I started working there, the Troubles already had a major impact on the social and environmental landscape.

Streets of bricked-up housing and empty shop fronts, a mix of Troubles-induced decay amidst urban renewal planning. Twentieth century housing was to replace old dwellings with their outside toilets built during the Victorian industrial boom time of the city. A time when Belfast was world famous for linen, rope-making and shipbuilding.

A second generation of children born during the Troubles was growing up, many in single-parent homes, the fathers imprisoned for paramilitary activity or on the run. Throwing stones at police and army vehicles was a common pastime for these children.

One period I particularly remember is the time of the 'supergrass' trials, when families moved overnight because of the fear of being named or of being arrested. They just seemed to disappear.

Health and educational needs were not a priority; health appointments were missed if a prison visit was due or travel to the clinic involved going through 'the other side's' territory.

Many of the families had the same problems as those faced in any other areas of social deprivation, with high levels of unemployment and poor educational achievement. However, the Troubles and their impact on this part of Belfast were never far away.

The 'peace wall' divided the two communities between the Catholic Falls and Protestant Shankill. Its huge gates opened by day to let traffic through and closed at night to prevent sectarian gun attacks. The neighbourhoods on each side of this wall not only had to contend with sectarian attack, but frequently endured feuding between different factions within their own community.

Finding addresses became an art as one manoeuvred through demolished areas and streets with their names blacked out. So many stressed mothers, most trying to do the best for their children.

When the first ceasefire was declared in 1994 I drove up the Falls Road. This was an historic occasion. People were on the streets cheering. I drove past the Royal Victoria Hospital and reflected on my nursing career. I had not known what it was like to work in peacetime and now, perhaps, I would. What would it all mean for community nursing? And what would the future hold for all the families living in this area?

I remembered many of the patients I nursed during my student years... security personnel with their brain injuries, including depressed fractures, shells of human beings, many still alive but totally dependent on carers. Injured paramilitary suspects; the knee-capped; civilians damaged through bomb blast; the Red Lion victims admitted to the ward three weeks into my first placement. What had become of all these patients and their families? I remembered the injuries but no faces, no names... so many buried memories.

Now there was hope for a better tomorrow, moods slowly changed and a feeling of optimism began to ripple through the community: a real 'feel-good factor' was all around. There was hope of investment and financial support for the local community. Then the Drumcree conflict flared.

Up went the barricades and roadblocks, getting home was subject to delay and fears grew that trouble would again explode onto the streets. Community nursing in many areas of the province had to start contingency planning to ensure all vulnerable patients would receive the night time care they required. Evening services were dependent on staff knowing alternative routes around the district. Rioting, mostly by youths, started along the peace line. For some staff it was all too much for their family and requests were made to redeploy.

Evening clinics were disrupted and some staff were unable to get home and so had to 'board out' for the evening. Each year at the same time, contingency planning had to start again and this had to be communicated in addition to normal duties.

Then at last came the year there was no need to plan, no barricades, no riots and uneventful journeys home. This was peace.

But in 2001 came the Holy Cross stand-off at Ardoyne, North Belfast. Community services disrupted yet again. This time the pressure fell on school nurses to support an increased number of children suffering from nocturnal enuresis and other disturbed behaviours as a result of this incident. Parents were given advice in groups. Many vulnerable people were caught up in this dispute including those with learning disability and mental health conditions.

As in all outbreaks of unrest, the resulting emotional and physical impact will remain with many people for the foreseeable future. Even today when rioting flares up, my thoughts go out to all the nurses and their colleagues who are doing their best to maintain normal services in very difficult circumstances. **"**

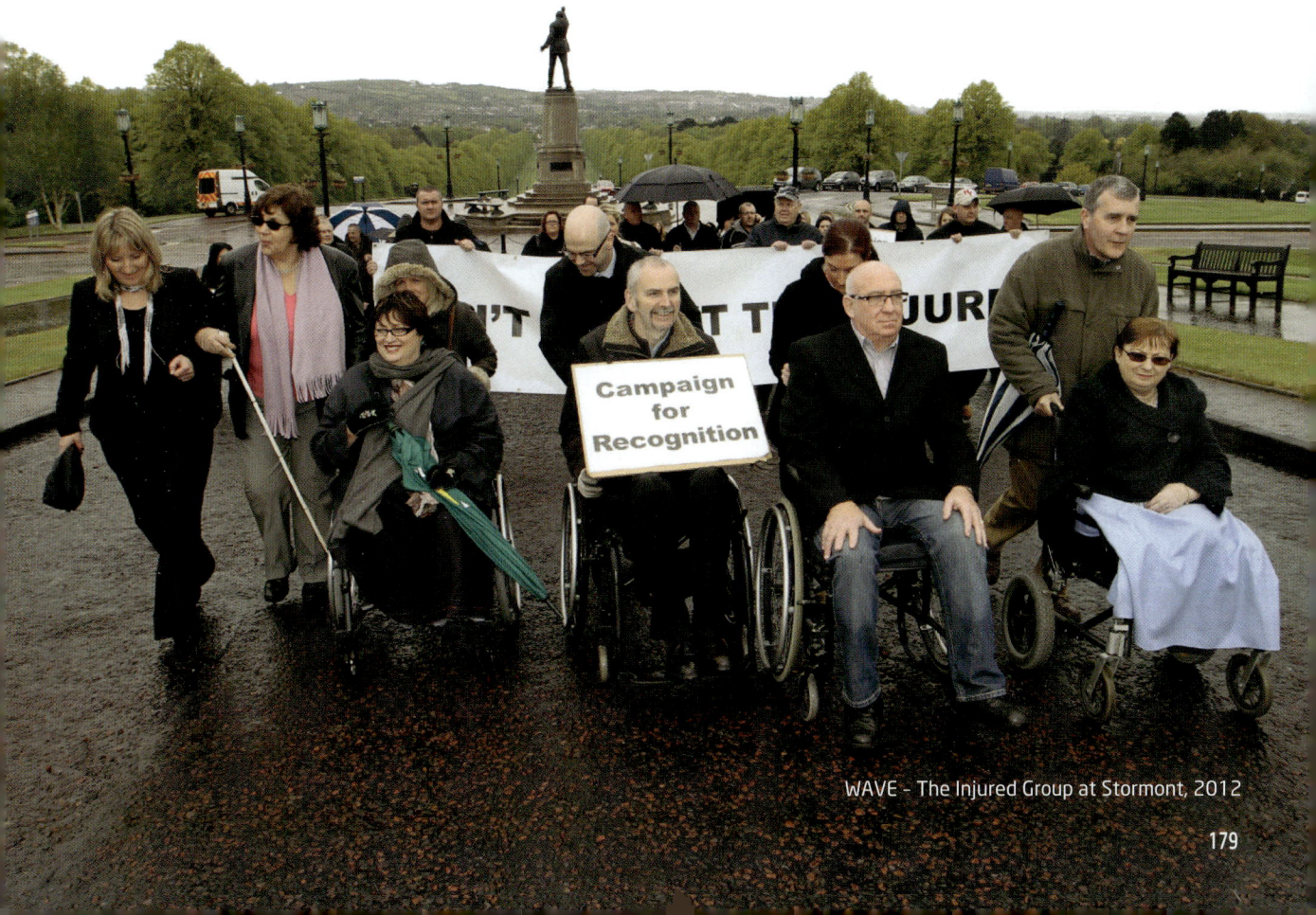

Family impact

“ *I have nursed bombers in the community and hospital, and nursed them 105%. It was very difficult for me because my husband was shot dead in the course of his work.*”

Staff Nurse

WAVE - The Injured Group at Stormont, 2012

"Daddy I love you so much." These were the last words Marie Wilson spoke to her father Gordon Wilson after the bomb exploded at the Enniskillen cenotaph on Remembrance Sunday, 1987.

Marie Wilson was the youngest nurse to be killed during the Troubles. Colleagues recalled her love of nursing and how she endeared herself to all those who knew her and worked with her.

Marie posthumously received the title Woman of Courage at a ceremony on February 8 1988 at the Dorchester Hotel, London, and her father collected the award on her behalf. He had made world headlines after the bomb when he said:

"I bear no ill will. I bear no grudge; that sort of talk is not going to bring her back to life. She was a great wee lassie. She loved her profession. And she's dead."

As the stories for this book were gathered, nurses spoke fondly of colleagues who had been killed in bombings. Jessie Johnston and Georgina Quinton were retired nurses who died in the Enniskillen bomb and Elizabeth McElhinney, a retired nurse from Altnagelvin, was killed in the Claudy bomb.

The number of nurses killed as a direct result of the Troubles is not known. A number of male nurses who were part-time members of security forces were shot as they arrived for work. And some nurses remembered colleagues who had to leave the profession following injuries that were the result of violence.

Northern Ireland is a small community and nurses are a key part of it. Some who had a family member in the security forces recalled their fear of this being discovered by colleagues. "Trust no one" was their mantra. Other nurses had family members who were associated with paramilitary organisations and were fearful of this becoming known. Many nurses suffered bereavement losing a family member to bombs or bullets. Some lost more than one relative and yet most returned to work.

Many nurses spoke of their fear of seeing a family member arrive in hospital as a casualty of the violence.

A shock in A&E

❝On 5 December 1971 I was a staff nurse on duty in Daisy Hill Hospital, Newry. I was asked to go to the A&E department to assist with patients who were admitted following 'gunshot wounds'.

On entering a cubicle I saw my sister lying on a trolley and my sister-in-law sitting on a chair. Both were very shocked and my sister had obvious abdominal injuries as she was bleeding. They explained that they had been caught in crossfire.

It was evident that the staff were not aware that these were my relatives. The evening passed in a daze and I left the hospital at midnight, returned at 3am to enquire about my sister as we didn't have a phone, then I came on duty at 8am. My sister made a good recovery following surgery and a lengthy stay in hospital.❞

Question: why the secrecy?
Answer: to protect!

"It was not until I reflected on the past Troubles that I asked myself the question, why was I so secret about my personal life?

I was well known as a caring nurse, a good nurse, but my personal life as a wife, a mother, a daughter, and a sister was only minimally discussed with nursing colleagues. That part of my life was protected.

As a girl I lived most of my life in the countryside. Our neighbours were Protestant. I went to a Protestant school. Later we moved nearer the town and I went to a 'mixed' school. It was only then that I had contact with other young people who were of a different religion to me. Was there a difference? Not really, we sat together, we talked to each other.

Then I went nursing. I had good friends from both religious denominations. The Troubles started a few years later just after I married. My first child was three years old and my second around nine months. I remember seeing the tanks coming in. It was scary – this was real! I felt so protective towards my children, but little did I know that the Troubles would last all through their childhood, into their adolescence and even into their early married lives.

After the army appeared, the Troubles over time became worse. Two of our neighbours were killed in separate incidents. We knew them well. One was only a young man. He had spent much of his youth in our home. The other was a father and a good friend of my father. I saw the effect these killings had on my parents.

My mother was in the Red Cross and she was one of the first at the scene of our young friend's killing. I saw the hurt and confusion that it caused. The next day I heard other nurses discussing the incident… I said little… I reflected on my father's words: 'How can they do this to their neighbour?'

It was better to say little. To protect my parents who lived in this area. To protect my brothers who were in the security forces. To protect my husband who worked alongside them. We never knew who could be next. It was better not to say too much, better not to give too much away. As a nurse I was used to dealing with trauma and crisis, but I had never had to deal with personal feelings of uncertainty like this before. I was a nurse, a good nurse, they told me that… the policeman, the gunman, the man and woman in the street that I nursed. It made no difference, they were my patients and I was their nurse.

I was five months pregnant when the Troubles directly hit our family. It was when my young sibling was caught in gunfire by the army – not on the street but in a restaurant having coffee with a friend. We were away on holiday when my brother phoned with the news. Things were critical. Now I was an anxious relative not only a nurse. What were the survival chances? How would my parents cope? Many, many questions, many fears. Fears about the future that I could not at that time share with my parents. I must not worry them. I must protect them.

It was a long haul for my sibling, a long caring process, a long rehabilitation. I did not work at that hospital. I didn't know the staff. I was a nurse but I felt like a stranger in that hospital. Why was I so out of my comfort zone? How many other nurses have felt like this during the Troubles?

Many nurses had family members who were injured or killed – did they feel like this? We were used to caring for others, protecting our families. It was second nature to us, but perhaps in times like this, we also needed to be 'cared for' as a relative and not just as a nurse.

As the Troubles continued, my parents decided to move to another part of the country far from the troubled area. I helped them to pack up and move. It must have been so hard for them. They had lived there all their lives, but they knew it would be better to move, it would be easier for my brothers to come home.

Life went on. We wanted our children to have as normal a life as possible. We spoke little about the Troubles in front of them. We chose to live in a 'mixed' area, to send our children to 'mixed' social activities, but we automatically looked under our car for a bomb before we got into it. We worried when they were teenagers and they wanted to go to discos… what if there is a bomb tonight in that area…?

I was a nurse, but I was a mother, a wife and a family member. One person, two roles: professional and personal. On reflection, the Troubles had a huge impact on both of those roles.**"**

The loss of a brother

A student nurse recalls…

"My mother had died and there was only my elderly father and brother at home on the farm. I was a third-year student at the Royal Victoria Hospital.

I would go home every third day or at weekends to do the chores. One night, arriving back at the nurses' accommodation at the Towers I was horrified to see my dog in the car boot – I tied him up in a sheltered part of the roof outside the flats. I went out there and found the roof was full of armed soldiers, which frightened me. My brother had to make the long journey at night through dangerous countryside and dangerous parts of Belfast to come and fetch my dog and take him home.

One day I was at home with a friend. It was about 6 pm. My brother and his friend had been at a ploughing match. I had set the table for their tea and my brother sat in our father's usual chair and his friend in my brother's seat. I was upstairs when I heard the gunfire. Running down the stairs I found my brother had been shot. His brain was blown out; in panic I tried to put some back, even though I knew it was useless. I felt I had to do something.

I don't know how I coped at the time – there was only me and my father. I had to give up work and hopes of doing midwifery training to run the farm. My father never got over it. I was given great support from the nursing administration in the Royal and from friends and my nursing crowd. One of the domestics from my ward sent me a card and I appreciated this as she was of a different religion from me and would have had to go to some trouble to get my address.

No one was ever held responsible for my brother's murder. He was not in any organisation or part of the security forces. There were a number of similar killings of farmers' sons along the border. I tried to find out who had been responsible but nobody wanted to know – I was just one person with no back-up.

I hit a difficult time much later… you can go different ways… I tried to continue to trust and not feel bitter; I know there are good people about. I think I put some dreadful memories in a box at the back of my head. I would be too afraid to open it. **"**

The dread

An off-duty sister remembers…

"On July 21 1972, which came to be known as Bloody Friday, I had a half-day and was driving down to visit my parents in Enniskillen, oblivious to what was happening in Belfast as I did not have a car radio. When I arrived, my parents were standing on the doorstep watching for me, sick with anxiety that I might have been caught up in one of the many bomb explosions. This brought home to me what it must have been like to be one of the many families who had relatives working in high-risk areas… the dread they must have experienced many times when reports of shooting and bombs were in the news. **"**

Off duty

"Days off, a time to relax and get away from the demands of nursing. Smiling faces heading out the door: 'See you in two days, I'm off,' a remark that always prompted the response: 'Lucky you, enjoy.'**

Was it really off duty? For many of us it was just the second shift. For me it was the start of the role of wife and mother – all the normal sort of stuff really. Although not quite of course – nothing in Northern Ireland was 'normal'. Being off duty meant being mum with all that that entails – the school run, sports events, homework, responding to 99 questions: 'Where's my football boots?', 'Where's my PE kit?'' and so it went on. Amid the mayhem of life in the Troubles you tried to maintain some degree of normality. But 'normality' meant living in a shadow, a hidden world where nothing is what it appears.

When mum always checks underneath the car before she lets the kids out of the house. 'Mum, why don't you just get the exhaust fixed, then you wouldn't have to check if it's still there all the time?… Or: My friend's mum always hangs the washing on the line outside, not in the attic like you do… Everyone else's mum lets them answer the door or the phone. Why can't we?… Why do we have to practise getting out of the house if there's a fire every week?… Mum, why don't you ever give anyone our address or phone number?… Why do you sit in the dark in the living room so late into the night?… and …Mum, why does Daddy not come home for days and days?'

Why? **"**

My nursing journey: the Troubles and beyond

A nurse, now a chief executive officer, working in the voluntary sector tells her story...

❝As a child I was very fortunate growing up in the idyllic County Down countryside near Spa and I ran free, without any fear. However I spent many summers during the late 1970s and early 1980s at my grandmother's home on the Fermanagh/Cavan border, and the atmosphere there was totally different.

I remember my granny telling me it wasn't like home. You had to be careful and the lights had to be off at night as you never knew who could be outside. Many a morning she woke to find windows in her outhouses missing, broken by an army night patrol looking to see what was in there. The ever-present field patrols and roadside checkpoints added to the tension and there was always the sense of hidden danger lurking.

Granny's sense of fear was well founded. In 1974 a bomb in a milk churn was planted close to her house. She stubbornly refused to leave and the milk churn lay beside the house for days. Concerned for her safety my uncle, with the help of a neighbour, attached a wire to the bomb and pulled it out into the middle of an adjoining field. The bomb disposal squad came later that day. Sadly, the bomb exploded prematurely and the bomb disposal officer was killed instantly. He was 32 years old and the father of three children. My granny talked about finding bits of his belongings, clothing and skin on the barbed wire fences and trees when she went out to look after her cattle. She spoke quietly but her message was clear: man's inhumanity to man would achieve nothing other than heartache."

Beginning my nursing career

From a young age I wanted to be a nurse. My mother had nursed and my grandmother, while never formally trained, was looked on as the woman to go to when anyone was sick or dying. I became part of the October 1987 intake to the Royal Victoria Hospital.

As a 19-year-old student in theatres, I remember a young soldier coming in with leg and facial injuries caused by shrapnel from a road-side bomb. He was also 19 and we shared the same birthday. This was his second visit to theatre as he had already had one leg amputated and the surgical team wanted to determine if they could save his other leg. Sadly they could not and it too was amputated.

As the student I was given the job of carrying his limb up to a porter waiting at the theatre doors. I vividly remember that walk. The leg felt so heavy and no matter how I carried it, the bone kept touching my leg through the bag. I found it so profoundly sad that the 19 year old who lay in theatre would eventually wake several days later in intensive care with such permanent and debilitating injuries, while I, at the same age, was celebrating my birthday with friends and enjoying all that it entailed.

The camaraderie among the students and staff prevailed even in the most extreme circumstances. The fact that the Troubles were happening around us was never far from our thoughts and even when off duty, the impact was ever present. Whether you lived outside the hospital or in the nurses' accommodation in the three towers at the entrance to the Royal, security alerts were a regular occurrence.

The army had a lookout post on the top floor of Victoria Tower, which was shot at on a regular basis. I remember being woken from a deep post-night shift sleep by this almighty banging and being told to get out as there was a security alert.

Nursing in the Troubles didn't just throw up medical challenges. On occasion you were confronted with moral dilemmas too. I was asked to 'special' (provide one-to-one care) to a young man who had been injured while planting a bomb that had caused loss of life. He was in the security wing. He had been blinded and had other injuries.

I talked to him and read him the paper, which was hard, as the first four pages were about what he had done. One of the bank nurses remarked later that she couldn't have looked after him. I reflected afterwards whether it was right that my colleague could put her opinions of the patient, and what he had done, before her professional duty to take care of him. I didn't know that bank nurse, but she may well have had a story of loss or family injury, and the challenge of looking after this young man may have been too great.

Nurses were by no means immune to the impact of the Troubles. Some were injured or killed, others lost relatives or had family members who were maimed. Many struggled with the impact of what they had witnessed and there was often a reluctance to talk about the unspeakable for fear of the consequences. This was the sad reality of how people lived.

Moving to the voluntary sector
It was only in 1995 when I came to WAVE, a trauma centre set up to cater for those bereaved or injured as a result of the Troubles, that I had a real sense of the long-term devastation caused for so many people. I had been blind to the scale of loss, injury and isolation experienced by individuals and their families. While the surgical and nursing teams at the Royal became world-renowned for their pioneering surgery and treatment of bomb, shooting and blast injuries, little or no attention had been given to developing treatments for the psychological trauma suffered by those bereaved and injured. This was reflected in the testimonies of many who came to WAVE for help and support.

One of the first people I met was a woman called Myrtle Hamilton. Myrtle had been widowed in 1974. She was a mother to two little girls and four months pregnant with her third child when her husband was murdered. I was struck by the fact that her husband had been killed on the same weekend as the bomb disposal officer in Fermanagh. Incidents 150 miles apart yet connected. There were a series of 'tit for tat murders' that weekend, as individuals were killed indiscriminately in retaliation for murders in the other community. Northern Ireland is small and inevitably cases were connected. These connections became apparent to me as my work in WAVE progressed, and highlighted the difficulties individuals had in talking about what had happened as they tried to gauge where the information might end up.

Myrtle made it very clear to me from the outset that she was volunteering in WAVE to help support other people rather than seeking help as a victim/survivor, and she and I worked together for over 12 years. A central tenet of WAVE's work was to offer support and assistance to those bereaved and injured by the Troubles, regardless of religious, political or cultural belief. I worked with Myrtle and others to develop a range of support services that were offered across the community. While delivering these support services what struck me was the sense of isolation felt by almost all those who came to us for help. This isolation was compounded when their loved one had been murdered or maimed by what was perceived to be 'their own' community. The silence around these cases was often deafening.

'Please don't forget about us'

I discovered very early on that political developments that can be perceived as positive or negative are often the catalyst in making individuals come forward for assistance. From the mid-1990s and the signing of the Good Friday Agreement, the number of victims/survivors seeking help increased. Many had lost limbs or sight, others had shrapnel or gunshot wounds and many had injuries that were not visible.

The sense of being hidden within society was mentioned by many. This lack of recognition was compounded by the absence of any official list of those injured and the fact that several government reports had not referred to their specific needs. One of the first women that I met was Jennifer McNern who, along with her sister and a number of others, had been badly injured in the Abercorn explosion in 1972. Jennifer and a number of others formed an injured support group, whose central message was 'please don't forget about us'.

I began seeking funding to undertake a research study into the needs of those injured in the Troubles and their families. After several false dawns this was finally achieved and the findings of the research report became the cornerstone of a Campaign for Recognition led by Jennifer and others for the injured and their families. This campaign has taken them to Westminster, The Dail and Stormont.

The 'disappeared'

Just after I joined WAVE I met a woman called Margaret McKinney whose son had 'disappeared' during the Troubles. The day we met she told me about her son's abduction, along with the story of another young man 16 years previously. She finished by saying: 'Love, I don't know what you can do for me' and in truth I didn't know myself. I started to work with Margaret on the issue of the disappeared, gradually meeting members of the other families who were affected in the same way. It was an issue that was very much hidden and the families had often been threatened. Trust was therefore a major consideration.

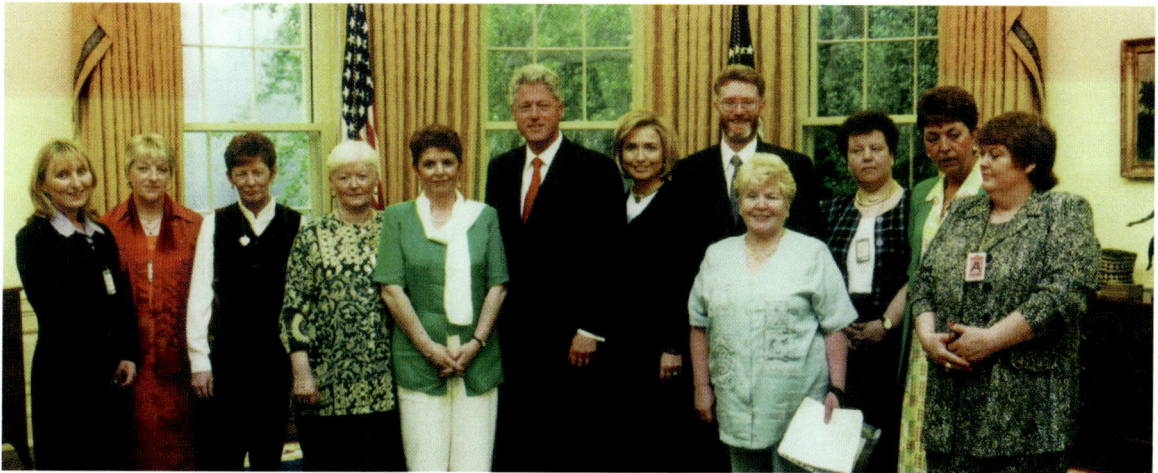

WAVE Group at the White House, 1998

We sought to get the issue out into the open. The campaign took us to the White House in the United States, the House of Commons in London and the Dail in Dublin, and it resulted in the establishment of an Independent Commission for the Location of Victims' Remains (ICLVR) in 1999. The commission acted as a conduit for gathering information, which was treated as privileged on the location of the disappeared, from those who did not wish to be identified. The search process commenced fairly quickly and many of the families were stunned to find that their loved ones had been taken over the border and were buried in the south of Ireland. Whilst a number of the bodies have been found, there are still seven families waiting for their loved ones to be brought home.

So the work continues.

Moving forward

Throughout my time at WAVE my nursing background has been invaluable. It allowed me to empathise with those who needed help and to work as part of a team, whose combined strengths have lifted WAVE from a small Belfast-based group to a Northern Ireland-wide victim/survivor support group.

I think of my grandmother often. Her assertion that man's inhumanity to man would achieve nothing but heartache has resonance each day. Every new referral received by WAVE is testament to this. I have been privileged and humbled as a nurse to work with some of those who have borne the brunt of the Troubles, both physically and psychologically. It is vital that we continue to support them as we move forward together in a shared future. **"**

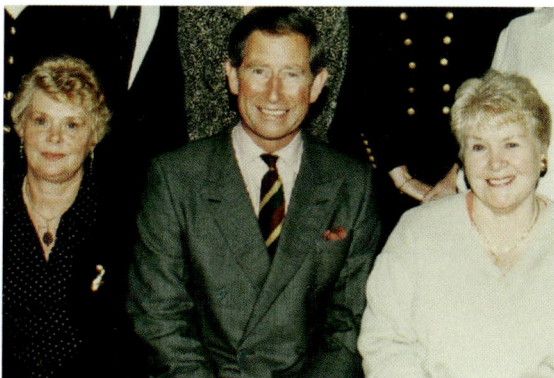

WAVE - Myrtle Hamilton and Margaret McKinney with Prince Charles

Footnote

When the History of Nursing Network in Northern Ireland began this project, the advice received from the author and journalist Alf McCreary was: "If you don't tell your story nobody will, your information and anecdotes will go with you. Your stories will be of interest to other nurses and the general public."

The history group hopes that these stories are of interest and have given a glimpse of the impact that the Troubles had on nurses who had to deal with unpredictable and traumatic situations.

Even today some nurses still have flashbacks of the horrific injuries they saw. Others find some memories too difficult to deal with; they cannot speak of them and have buried them deep inside.

As we met with nurses from across the province, all expressed the hope that those dark days would never return. As one nurse put it:

"How could we have done this to each other? How did things get to that? I lost my teenage years. I don't want my children or grandchildren to go through what I have experienced."

References for statistical and historical data (page viii)

1. Healing Through Remembering (2006) A Day of Private Reflection: Discussion Paper and Proposal. Healing Through Remembering, Belfast.

2. Northern Ireland Statistics and Research Agency. www.nisra.gov.uk

3. McKittrick D, Kelters S, Feeney B, Thornton C, McVea D (2007) Lost Lives. Mainstream Publishing, Edinburgh. (Updated using the Conflict Archive on the Internet (CAIN) http://cain.ulster.ac.uk/issues/violence/deaths2007draft.htm)

4. Conflict Archive on the Internet (CAIN), RUC/PSNI statistics: Table NI-SEC-05: Persons injured (number) due to the security situation in Northern Ireland (only), 1969 to 2003. Available at http://cain.ulster.ac.uk/ni/security.htm#05. Number is limited to injuries in Northern Ireland.

5. Conflict Archive on the Internet (CAIN), RUC/PSNI statistics: Table NI-SEC-06: Security related incidents (number) in Northern Ireland (only), shootings, bombings, and incendiaries, 1969 to 2003. Available at http://cain.ulster.ac.uk/ni/security.htm#06. Number is limited to shootings in Northern Ireland.

6. Fay M-T, Morrissey M, Smyth M (1999) Northern Ireland's Troubles: The Human Costs. Pluto Press, London.

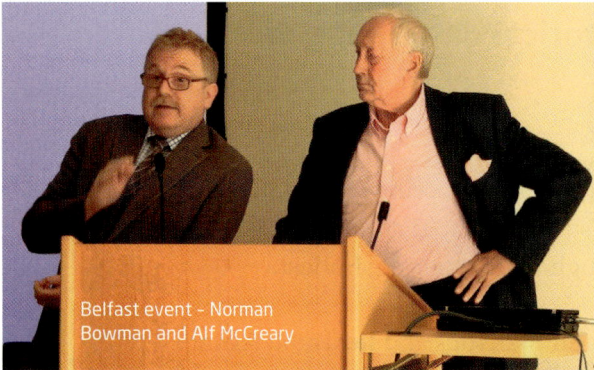
Belfast event – Norman Bowman and Alf McCreary

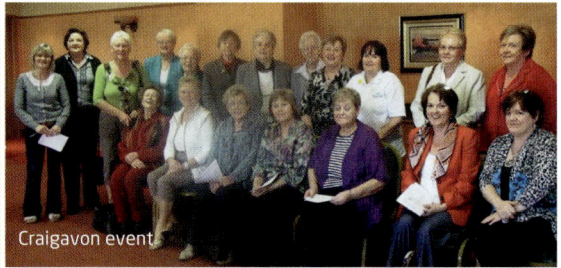
Craigavon event

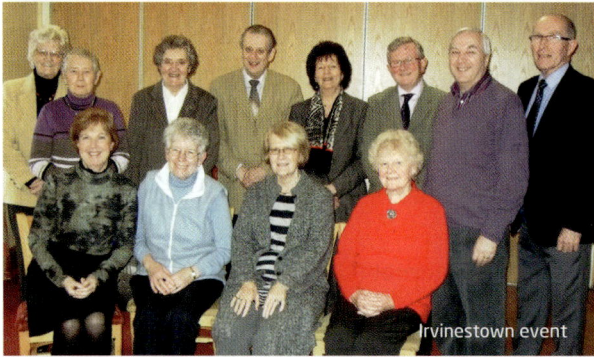
Irvinestown event

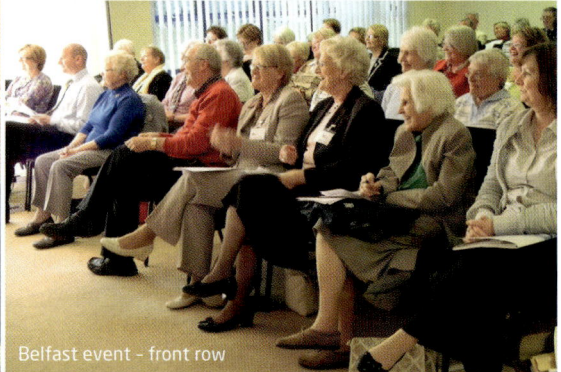
Belfast event – front row

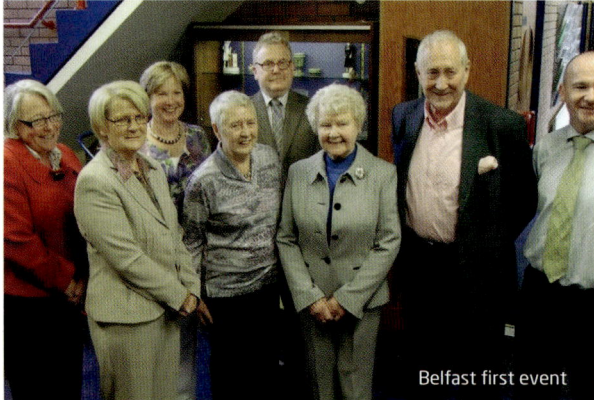
Belfast first event

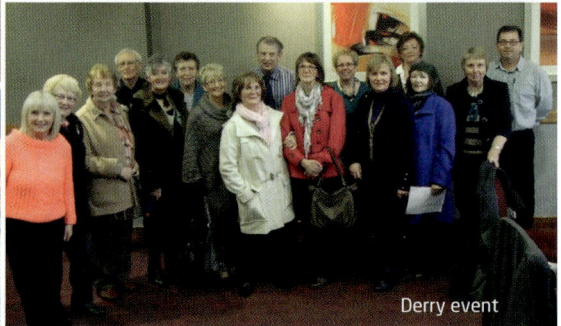
Derry event

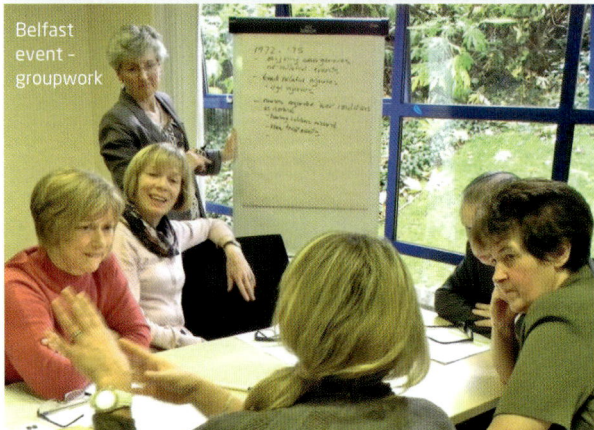
Belfast event – groupwork

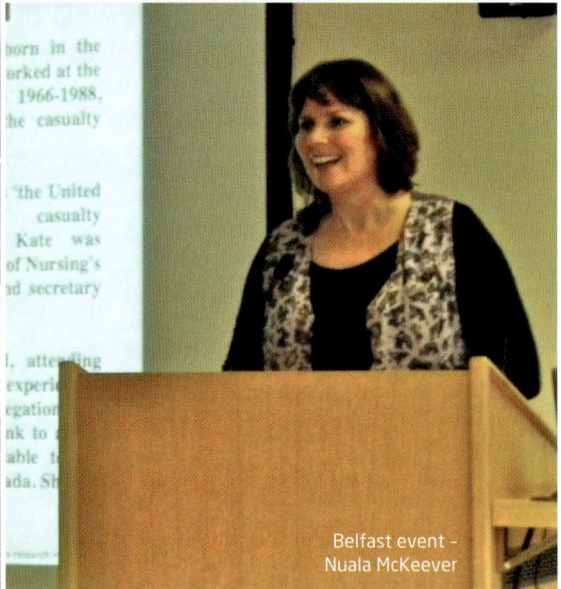
Belfast event – Nuala McKeever

APPENDIX A

How our nursing stories were gathered

In 2011 when the History Group decided to gather stories about nursing during the Troubles, a first priority was to gauge the level of support in the profession as nurses are notoriously "backward about coming forward". More significantly, it was the fact that most nurses who had worked through the late 1960s and early 1970s had retired and might not be reached easily. Even if they could be, they might not wish to recount events dating back some 30 or 40 years.

To get the project started a workshop was planned inviting nurses who had worked in any capacity, at any time, through the Troubles to come and tell their story.

Any concerns about undertaking the project were quickly dispelled when, following notice of the event, some 60 nurses gathered at the RCN headquarters in Belfast on 24 May 2011. This was a very encouraging response and, importantly, it was clear from conversations on the day that many of those attending had heard about the event from other nurses.

At an early stage in planning the seminar it was considered important to encourage the more reticent to tell their stories. To this end Alf McCreary, the well known Northern Ireland journalist and author with a special interest in the Troubles (notably "Survivors" published in 1976), was invited to head up the day. His brief was to share his journalistic experience and comment on the process of gathering and presenting the kind of stories we had in mind.

An important feature of the day was five interviews conducted by Alf who spoke to nurses who had worked in different capacities and locations across the decades. These "interviewees" had been identified beforehand on the basis that they represented a broad spectrum of nursing ranging from community and mental health nursing to accident and emergency, theatre and ward nursing. The interviewees had also worked in different hospitals and community locations across the province and during various decades of the Troubles. This worked well and the stories told stimulated debate and encouraged recollections from many of the audience.

Another very useful element of the day was a photographic presentation of historical material gathered from media and personal photographs, and other archive material, made accessible by a retired nurse. These provided an evocative and often poignant backdrop to the day and added sometimes forgotten detail to the broader background of the stories being told.

At the end of the day as delegates headed home there were many encouraging comments and strong support for the project. This initial event was judged a success both by the committee and the majority of those attending. Nurses clearly had plenty of stories to tell.

A second event organised along similar lines was also well supported. On this occasion the event was facilitated by Nuala McKeever, local actor, comedienne and journalist. Reminiscences on this second day ranged across the same broad spectrum of experiences as at the first event. Evident again was the capacity of nurses to see some humour in all but the most testing situations.

At both events participants were given some guidance in the development and presentation of the stories. Notes provided were not intended to be directive but simply aimed to generate debate and achieve the best from the limited amount of time available. The notes were also intended to help nurses who might want to submit their story at a later date.

On both days participants quickly warmed to their task and discussions could have continued much longer than the day allowed. Once people relaxed and listened to reminiscences, they contributed their own stories.

In the following months a number of more local events were organised in Derry/ Londonderry, Irvinestown, Fermanagh, and Craigavon, Armagh, all in an effort to ensure the widest coverage of the province. These events, by nature of their location, were attended by a smaller number of nurses. Meetings were informal and less structured but were informative and again generated much debate and enthusiasm from those who attended. Again it was evident that there was a strong cathartic effect in the airing of stories, not just on the part of the storyteller but on the gathered audience of the day.

Overall the five events generated directly or indirectly the personal stories and reminiscences that form the heart of this book. "Word of mouth" following the organised events was a major factor in securing many more of the stories included. Some were sent by email and some are from nurses now based outside Northern Ireland. Together they give what we, the History of Nursing Network in Northern Ireland, hope is a picture that does justice to the profession and to the many, many nurses who worked through these troubled times.

APPENDIX B

Chronology of events referenced in the stories told

12-14 August 1969
Battle of the Bogside
Rioting erupts between
residents and police lasting
for several days.

13-15 August 1969
Troubles in Derry/
Londonderry overflow
to Belfast where rioting
erupts and streets are set
alight in West Belfast.

15 August 1969
British troops deployed
following unrest in Derry/
Londonderry and Belfast.

25 May 1971
Springfield Road Police
Station bomb.
One man killed,
27 injured.

August 9 1971
Internment
Suspected terrorists
detained under Special
Powers Act (Northern
Ireland) 1922.

4 December 1971
McGurk's Bar bomb.
15 killed, men, women and
children; 17 injured.

11 December 1971
Balmoral Furniture Company
bomb on the Shankill Road.
Two adults and two children
killed.

30 January 1972
Bloody Sunday.
Thirteen men killed, 13
injured (one later died).

4 March 1972
Abercorn Restaurant bomb.
Two women killed, 130
injured.

30 May 1972
Springfield Road Police
Station bomb.
One man killed, six injured.

21 July 1972
Bloody Friday.
Nine men, women and
children killed; 130 injured.

31 July 1972
Operation Motorman.
Army operation to remove
barricades erected to block
access to areas controlled by
paramilitary organisations.

31 July 1972
Claudy bombing.
Nine men, women and
children killed; 30 injured.

15-28 May 1974
Ulster Workers' Council
strike. A Loyalist/Unionist
strike to oppose the political
solution that established a
power-sharing government.
A total of 39 people killed
during this period, 33 in
Dublin and Monaghan
bombings.

5 January 1976
Kingsmill massacre.
Eleven men shot, one
survived.

17 February 1978
La Mon Restaurant/Hotel
Bomb
Twelve men and women
killed, 30 injured.

31 August 1979
Warrenpoint ambush.
Eighteen men killed, six
injured.

6 December 1982
Droppin' Well bomb,
Ballykelly.
Seventeen men and women
killed, 30 injured.

4 November 1983
Ulster Polytechnic,
Jordanstown, County
Antrim. Two killed,
33 injured.

8 November 1987
Enniskillen Poppy Day bomb.
Twelve men and women
killed, 63 injured.

16 March 1988
Milltown cemetery attack.
Three men killed,
60 injured.

20 August 1988
Ballygawley bus bombing.
Eight men killed, 28 injured.

2 November 1991
Musgrave Hospital bomb.
Two men killed, 11 injured
including two children.

5 February 1992
Sean Graham's Bookmakers
shootings.
Five killed, nine injured.

23 October 1993
Shankill bomb.
Ten men and women killed,
57 injured.

30 October 1993
Greysteel massacre.
Eight men and women
killed, 13 injured.

31 August 1994
First IRA ceasefire.
It ended on February 9 1996
with a bomb in London's
Docklands.
Two killed, 100 people
injured.

19 July 1997
Second IRA ceasefire.

10 April 1998
Good Friday or Belfast
Agreement.
A landmark political
agreement in the peace
process.

15 August 1998
Omagh bomb.
Twenty nine men, women
and children killed,
including unborn twins,
220 or more injured.

July 1995-1998
Drumcree conflict – dispute
over the route of an annual
parade held during the first
week of July. Several
hundred injured during
violence accompanying the
disputed parade.

October 2006
St Andrew's Agreement.
Northern Ireland Assembly
restored following talks
between British and Irish
governments and Northern
Ireland political parties.

APPENDIX C

Glossary

1921 Ireland was partitioned into two distinct territories: the Republic of Ireland and Northern Ireland (as part of the UK). Civil unrest flared between Catholic and Protestant communities in Northern Ireland.

ARDOYNE Residential area of North Belfast.

B SPECIALS Ulster Special Constabulary (now disbanded).

BALLYMURPHY Residential area of West Belfast.

BALLYOWEN Residential area of West Belfast.

BOGSIDE Residential area of Derry/Londonderry.

BOMBAY STREET Residential area of West Belfast.

BOSTOCK HOUSE Resident nurses' accommodation on Royal Victoria Hospital site.

BROADWAY Residential area of West Belfast.

BROADWAY TOWERS One of three high-rise buildings between Protestant and Catholic areas at Broadway, Belfast. Opposite the rear exit of the Royal Hospitals complex, it provided accommodation for hospital staff.

CORRYMEELA Corrymeela Community, Ballycastle, was established before the Troubles in 1965 and became a reconciliation centre for both sides of the community.

DELAYED PRIMARY SUTURE The surgical closure of a wound several days after the injury because the wound was initially too contaminated to close.

DIVIS FLATS High-rise block of flats in the Republican area of West Belfast.

GARDA SIOCHÁNA The official Police Force in the Republic of Ireland.

GROSVENOR ROAD Residential area of West Belfast.

GROSVENOR TOWERS One of three high-rise buildings between Protestant and Catholic areas at Broadway, Belfast. Opposite the rear exit of the Royal Hospitals complex, it provided accommodation for hospital staff.

HOME OFFICE Nursing Administrative Officers, Royal Victoria Hospital.

HOSPITAL SERVICE RESERVES Volunteer workers.

KING BILLY Refers to William Prince of Orange, later King William III of Great Britain and Ireland, 1689-1702.

LA MON   A hotel and restaurant complex in Gransha, on the outskirts of Belfast. Scene of a major bomb blast on 17 February 1978. Twelve people killed and more than 30 injured.

MAZE/LONG KESH   A prison complex near Lisburn, County Down.

MUSGRAVE PARK HOSPITAL   Situated in Belfast, this specialist orthopaedic hospital also had a secure military wing.

MUSSON HOUSE   Residential accommodation on-site for student nursing staff at the Royal Victoria Hospital, Belfast. It also provided facilities for the School of Nursing.

NEW LODGE   Residential area of North Belfast.

PEACE LINE   A purpose-built high wall to separate/provide protection for two communities living side-by-side.

RED SISTER   Senior Ward Sister, Royal Victoria Hospital – identified by their red uniform dress.

ROSEMOUNT   Residential area of Derry/ Londonderry.

RUC   Royal Ulster Constabulary. Re-named as the Police Service of Northern Ireland (PSNI) in 2001.

SHANKILL   Residential area of West Belfast.

STORMONT   Official seat of government in Northern Ireland.

THE CREGGAN   Residential area of Derry/ Londonderry.

TIGER'S BAY   Residential area of North Belfast.

ULSTER WORKERS' STRIKE   Called by the Ulster Workers' Council in 1974 in protest against the Sunningdale Agreement, this brought down the power-sharing Executive at Stormont.

VICTORIA TOWERS   One of three high-rise buildings between Protestant and Catholic areas at Broadway, Belfast. Opposite the rear exit of the Royal Hospitals complex, it provided accommodation for hospital staff.

WAVE TRAUMA CENTRE   A cross-community charity offering care and support to people bereaved, injured or traumatised as a result of the Troubles in Northern Ireland.

WEST OF THE BANN   A rural area in County Armagh, Northern Ireland, through which the River Bann flows.

WEST WING   Accessed from the main corridor at Royal Victoria Hospital. Ground-floor accommodated nursing administration offices. Other floors provided residential single rooms for nursing students, with some flats for senior nursing staff.

WITHERS   A ward in Musgrave Park Orthopaedic Hospital.

APPENDIX D

Abbreviations

ADNS   Assistant Director of Nursing Services

BCH   Belfast City Hospital

CAH   Craigavon Area Hospital

CPR   Cardiac pulmonary resuscitation, performed on patient in the event of cardiac arrest

CVP   Central venous pressure (line)

EENT   Eyes, ears, nose and throat Clinic

IRA   Irish Republican Army

IV lines   Intravenous lines for administration of drugs/fluids to patients

KOM   Knights of Malta

MIH   Mater Infirmorium Hospital

MPH   Musgrave Park Hospital

NI   Northern Ireland

NSU   Neurosurgical ward of Royal Victoria Hospital

PTS   Preliminary Training School, for student nurses

RBHSC   Royal Belfast Hospital for Sick Children

RCN   Royal College of Nursing

RICU   Respiratory intensive care unit

RMH   Royal Maternity Hospital, part of the Royal Victoria Hospital complex

RMN   Registered Mental Nurse

ROI   Republic of Ireland

RUC   Royal Ulster Constabulary

RVH   Royal Victoria Hospital (Belfast)

SEN   State Enrolled Nurse

SPG   Special Patrol Group (RUC)

SRN   State Registered Nurse

SOD   School of Dentistry, on the Royal Victoria Hospital site

UDR   Ulster Defence Regiment

UVF   Ulster Volunteer Force

APPENDIX E

Illustrations

At all of the events that the History of Nursing Network NI held to gather stories from nurses, all contributors were invited to send in any photographs they might have from this period of their career. The images in this book were submitted following this request.

Most of the photographs and newspaper cuttings have been supplied from the personal archive of Horace Reid, but there are also contributions from the following:

Attracta Bradley	Pamela McMillen
Anne Grant	Royal College of Nursing Northern Ireland
June Fulton	
Margaret Kelly	Western Health & Social Care Trust
Vera Hunniford	
John Hall	BBC Northern Ireland
Nora Patterson	Tyrone Constitution
Eric Wilkinson	Belfast Telegraph
Keith Graham	Daily Mirror
Laurie Jones	Belfast Newsletter
WAVE Trauma Centre	Irish News
Margaret McCambridge	The Times

All pictures are the copyright of the owners and should not be reproduced without the owner's permission.

A number of images have been acquired from Pacemaker Press, Victor Patterson Photographer, Joe Fox Photography, Eamon Melaugh and Press Association.

Pictures of Belfast Hospitals are the copyright of Belfast Health and Social Care Trust.

APPENDIX F

Acknowledgements

In bringing this collection of personal stories and memories together, we are grateful for the support and encouragement of many friends and colleagues.

Dr Peter Carter, Chief Executive and General Secretary of the Royal College of Nursing London, for approval to proceed with this project and release of funding from the Dr Mona Grey bequest.

Janice Smyth, Director of the RCN Northern Ireland, who has facilitated and encouraged us at all times and provided the resources of staff and facilities of the College.

History of Nursing Network Project Team and Committee who had the initial vision to gather the stories, and commitment and determination to carry this vision through to completion.

Kim Cobain, RCN administrator, without whose tireless support, dedication and hard work we could not have completed this book.

Professor Jean Orr CBE, Emeritus Professor of Nursing, Queen's University Belfast, who advised on, and edited, the many stories received.

Horace Reid, retired nurse and historian, who provided many photographs and newspaper reports dating from the early 1970s.

Mark Kelly and Jennifer McNern, from the injured group at WAVE Trauma Centre.

Ann Duff (née Fenton) and Lorna Finlay for provision of period uniform.

Professor Linda Johnston, School of Nursing and Midwifery, Queen's University Belfast, for the use of the clinical skills laboratory.

Alf McCreary, writer and journalist, who facilitated our first seminar, encouraged us and gave us the benefit of his experience.

Eric Wilkinson for the supply of photographs of his badge collection.

Dr Martin Melaugh of CAIN (Conflict Archive on the Internet) and Malcolm Sutton's 'An Index of Deaths from the Conflict in Ireland' for use of their statistical data.

Margaret Graham, Chair of HoN NI, for leading and ensuring completion of the book.

Fiona Carroll, Aisling Teague, Kevin Campbell and Victoria Graves for their assistance with the front cover shoot.

Fiona Bourne of the RCN Archives, Edinburgh, for help with sourcing materials and articles.

Index